AI-Powered
Fitness & Nutrition

How to Lose Weight, Boost Energy, and Optimize Health with Artificial Intelligence

Written by
Eric LeBouthillier

AcraSolution | 2025 1st Edition
www.acrasolution.com

Preface

Who This Book Is For

This book is written for anyone ready to follow a clear, structured path of growth. Whether you are a beginner seeking direction, a professional looking to refine your skills, or a creative mind searching for a framework to turn ideas into action, the chapters are designed to meet you where you are. If you want a guide that combines clarity with practicality, this book is for you.

What You Can Expect

Inside, you'll find a complete 12-chapter progression that walks you step by step from foundation to mastery. Each chapter is divided into multiple focused subtopics. Expect practical strategies, clear explanations, and actionable takeaways you can apply immediately. By the end, you'll have not only learned—but built the confidence to begin again, stronger and better prepared for what comes next.

Table of Contents

CHAPTER 1

The New Era of Fitness & Nutrition

Why Traditional Methods Often Fail

For decades, the health and fitness industry has been dominated by one-size-fits-all solutions: calorie-counting meal plans, rigid workout templates, and a belief that discipline alone determines results. But despite the explosion of gyms, apps, supplements, and coaching programs, obesity rates are still climbing, chronic disease is more common than ever, and millions of people are stuck in cycles of burnout, guilt, and frustration.

These aren't just personal failures. They're system failures — rooted in outdated, overly simplistic methods that ignore the complexity of human biology, psychology, and daily life. In today's world, where stress, sleep, metabolism, and even our microbiome play critical roles, relying on traditional approaches is like trying to navigate with a paper map in a GPS world.

The Problem With One-Size-Fits-All

Traditional programs assume that what works for one person will work for everyone. Whether it's the same 1,500-calorie diet or the same 12-week muscle-building plan, the old model treats humans like identical machines. But we're not machines — we're ecosystems. Each person's body responds differently based on genetics, hormones, mental state, and lifestyle.

This leads to a frustrating pattern: early progress followed by plateaus or reversals. People blame themselves for "falling off the wagon," but often it's the method — not the person — that failed.

Ignoring Data, Feedback, and Context

Another core issue with traditional methods is that they're static. They don't adapt to the individual's changing condition or behavior. Someone who just started a new stressful job, got poor sleep, or is recovering from illness may need very different nutritional or exercise support than someone in peak condition. But the old methods don't adjust — they assume consistency, even when life is anything but consistent.

Worse, many programs ask people to follow advice without ever explaining the *why*. Without understanding or feedback loops, motivation drops, adherence falls off, and long-term change becomes unlikely.

Outdated Science Meets Modern Marketing

Many traditional methods are still based on decades-old science — or worse, fads dressed up as science. Low-fat, high-carb diets were pushed for years despite mounting evidence that they weren't universally effective. The "no pain, no gain" mentality persists despite clear research on recovery, injury prevention, and sustainability.

Meanwhile, fitness and nutrition influencers flood social media with oversimplified advice, edited bodies, and performance-enhancing shortcuts — setting unrealistic expectations and confusing the public. The result is an industry where misinformation thrives and trust is fragile.

Real-World Example

What Happened
A mid-sized tech startup in Austin launched a company-wide wellness program to help reduce healthcare costs and boost productivity. They hired a consultant who implemented a generic 12-week fitness and diet plan, complete with weigh-ins, challenges, and leaderboards.

What Went Wrong
Within six weeks, participation dropped by 60%. Many employees felt judged by the weigh-ins, others reported injuries from workouts that were too aggressive, and some with specific health issues (e.g., diabetes, thyroid conditions) found the meal plan totally inappropriate. Morale declined, and by the end of the quarter, HR quietly shelved the program.

What We Learn From It
Health isn't one-dimensional. Without personalization, empathy, and adaptability, even well-funded wellness efforts can backfire. Success requires tools that *respond* to individual needs — not just impose blanket rules.

Common Pitfalls in Traditional Approaches

- **Static Plans:** No adjustment for changing stress, sleep, illness, or motivation
- **Overreliance on Willpower:** Ignores biological and psychological realities
- **Lack of Personalization:** Treats all bodies and goals the same
- **Punishment-Oriented Thinking:** Encourages guilt and shame over curiosity and progress
- **Unrealistic Standards:** Often modeled on elite athletes or influencers, not everyday people

Tactical Best Practices Moving Forward

- **Embrace Bio-Individuality:** Understand that everyone's body, schedule, and goals are different
- **Prioritize Adaptive Systems:** Use methods that evolve with the user's real-time data and feedback
- **Focus on Behavior, Not Just Outcomes:** Reinforce habits, routines, and emotional wins — not just weight loss or aesthetics

- **Encourage Understanding Over Obedience:** Educate users so they can make better decisions independently
- **Replace Judgment With Curiosity:** When progress stalls, ask *why*, not *what did you do wrong*

Checklist-Style Action Steps

1-Stop relying on generic diet or workout plans — they're rarely sustainable
2-Start tracking individual patterns (energy, sleep, stress, digestion) to see what *actually* works for you
3-Ask your coach or provider how your program will adapt as your needs evolve
4-Avoid programs that equate failure with lack of discipline
Seek tools that offer feedback and insight, not just rules to follow

Traditional methods aren't just ineffective — they're misaligned with the complexity of real life. What worked decades ago, or even a few years ago, can no longer meet the demands of today's bodies, minds, and schedules. Fitness and nutrition must evolve to become more human, more flexible, and far more intelligent.

That evolution is already underway — and it starts with AI.

The Rise of AI in Health and Wellness

Not long ago, fitness and nutrition advice followed a familiar pattern: follow this plan, eat these foods, do this workout, repeat. The expectation was that results would follow — if not, the blame often landed on the individual's "lack of willpower." But that model is being dismantled by something more sophisticated, more adaptive, and more forgiving: artificial intelligence.

AI isn't just making wellness more efficient — it's making it *smarter*. By analyzing data points that the human brain could never process at once — sleep patterns, heart rate variability, glucose levels, exercise output, mood, even subtle shifts in body temperature

— AI systems are giving people the ability to tailor their health strategy in ways we've never had access to before.

This isn't automation for the sake of convenience. It's intelligent orchestration of data, decisions, and outcomes — all built around *you*.

From Information Overload to Intelligent Guidance

Today's users are drowning in health information. Open your phone and you're one click away from 500 contradictory takes on fasting, protein intake, or the latest training split. The problem isn't a lack of knowledge — it's an inability to filter what applies to *your* body, your schedule, your goals.

This is where AI excels. Instead of adding more content to the noise, it personalizes and prioritizes based on what's happening *inside* your body in real time. AI can detect trends before you feel them. It can spot recovery deficits, predict plateaus, and recommend subtle changes that would be nearly impossible for a coach or user to see on their own.

For the first time, everyday people have access to decision-quality insight — not just advice.

A Shift From Coaching to Co-Piloting

In the traditional model, a personal trainer or nutritionist would assess your needs and design a plan. Then you'd try to follow it, adjusting as best you could when life inevitably changed. This put most of the burden on the user, and often left coaches blind to what was actually happening between sessions.

With AI, the model becomes collaborative. The system observes how your body is responding and *coaches itself* — nudging adjustments to workload, macronutrient balance, meal timing, or rest days. It's a living plan, not a static one. And it doesn't rely on willpower alone. It helps automate smart decisions so you don't have to constantly manage every detail.

The result is better adherence, faster feedback, and a drastically reduced risk of burnout or injury.

Real-Time Data Becomes Real-Time Decisions

Wearables, biometric scanners, and mobile trackers are now everywhere. But hardware without intelligent software is just noise. AI is what turns the firehose of raw metrics into actionable, human-centered recommendations.

Examples include:

- **Adjusting workouts based on recovery status** (e.g., lowering intensity when HRV is suppressed)
- **Dynamically changing macros** based on cycle tracking, glucose trends, or sleep debt
- **Providing proactive prompts** when daily movement is low or stress levels spike
- **Detecting illness onset** from small physiological shifts — before symptoms appear

Real-World Example

What Happened
A mid-30s executive in a high-stress role used to follow a strict low-carb diet and 6-day gym routine. Despite the effort, she was chronically tired, experienced frequent weight fluctuations, and struggled with sleep.

What Changed
She adopted an AI-enabled wellness system using a wearable ring and app. The platform monitored her recovery, cycle data, glucose, and workout output. The AI quickly identified a mismatch between her training load and recovery, and that her fasting windows were negatively impacting sleep. It shifted her to a carb-cycling model,

reduced intensity on poor recovery days, and added mindfulness prompts on high-stress workdays.

What We Learn From It
Her energy improved, sleep stabilized, and body composition shifted — not from harder work, but from *smarter feedback*. AI didn't replace her routine. It *refined* it, giving her back control through small, personalized tweaks based on real-time data.

Common Pitfalls to Avoid When Integrating AI

- **Chasing Metrics, Not Meaning**
  Data is seductive — but it's not all useful. The value lies in *interpreted* data, not raw numbers.
- **Over-Relying on Automation**
  AI should assist, not replace, your decision-making. Passive users get passive results.
- **Misaligned Tools**
  Not all AI systems are created equal. Many apps use the label but rely on rule-based logic, not true adaptive learning.
- **Ignoring Context**
  Even smart systems can misread your situation. You must still contextualize what the AI recommends.

Tactical Best Practices to Begin

- **Pair One Wearable With One Platform**
  Avoid tool overload. Start with a reliable combo that syncs well (e.g., Whoop + training app).
- **Track Only What You'll Use**
  Focus on 3–5 metrics that inform action: HRV, sleep, glucose, energy, movement.
- **Look for Pattern Recognition, Not Just Tracking**
  Choose tools that learn from *you*, not ones that just count steps or calories.
- **Combine AI Feedback With Human Intuition**
  AI knows the data. You know your life. Use both.

AI is no longer an experimental tool — it's becoming the foundation of next-generation health and fitness systems. By taking guesswork out of the equation and replacing it with continuous, personalized feedback, AI helps users build smarter, more sustainable wellness habits.

The real promise of AI isn't perfection. It's *progress without punishment.*

Next Steps
Next, we'll break down the **Core Benefits of AI for Fitness and Diet**, from personalization and recovery tracking to cognitive load reduction and long-term habit formation — all translated into clear takeaways you can apply immediately.

Core Benefits of AI for Fitness and Diet

The real power of AI in fitness and nutrition isn't in flashy features or futuristic interfaces. It's in its ability to solve problems that have frustrated people for decades: lack of personalization, information overload, inconsistent results, and unsustainable routines. When deployed correctly, AI can reduce the mental burden of staying healthy, guide better choices without constant guesswork, and support long-term change without requiring extreme effort.

Here's how.

1. Precision Personalization — At Scale

Generic advice is cheap. Personalized guidance, on the other hand, has always been expensive — traditionally requiring one-on-one access to coaches, dietitians, or doctors. AI changes that. By analyzing your biometric data, lifestyle inputs, and behavioral patterns, AI can deliver custom plans that adapt to your unique body and goals in real time.

Whether it's adjusting your protein intake based on muscle recovery, shifting your workout volume based on sleep quality, or recommending meal timing based on circadian patterns, AI turns impersonal programs into precision health.

This is especially important for:

- People with hormonal imbalances or metabolic issues
- Women with cycle-related fluctuations
- Shift workers or parents with irregular schedules
- Aging populations with changing recovery and strength curves

2. Real-Time Adaptability

Life changes — your health plan should too. Traditional programs fail because they don't adapt. If you're sick, stressed, under-slept, or traveling, your ability to train or follow a strict diet shifts. Most plans don't account for this. AI does.

It responds to your body in real time:

- **Low recovery today?** It downshifts your training load.
- **High stress?** It suggests parasympathetic activities like walks or mobility, not HIIT.
- **Consistently high glucose after breakfast?** It tweaks your macro ratios or food order.

These micro-adjustments keep you progressing without burning out. They remove the pressure to always "push through" and instead support smarter consistency.

3. Reduced Cognitive Load

One of the most underappreciated benefits of AI in wellness is the *reduction in mental effort*. Health decisions take up bandwidth — and in high-stress environments, decision fatigue sets in quickly.

What should I eat today? Should I work out? How hard should I train? What if I didn't sleep well?

AI removes those daily dilemmas by pre-filtering your options:

- Suggesting the right workout intensity based on recovery
- Recommending meals based on your current energy and blood sugar trends
- Reminding you to move if sedentary time builds up
- Nudging hydration or breathwork if your stress markers spike

The result? Less second-guessing, more doing — with less stress.

4. Early Detection and Prevention

Many health issues develop gradually. By the time symptoms are noticeable, damage is already underway. AI's ability to monitor patterns — not just numbers — gives it a head start on spotting trouble before you feel it.

Common use cases:

- **Detecting signs of overtraining** days before performance drops
- **Catching chronic stress trends** before they lead to burnout
- **Identifying blood sugar instability** that could trigger future metabolic issues
- **Tracking sleep quality deterioration** tied to hormonal or behavioral changes

This allows for proactive intervention instead of reactive treatment — something no static plan can deliver.

5. Habit Formation and Behavioral Nudging

Sustainable health comes from habits, not hacks. But building habits is hard — especially in busy lives. AI helps reinforce positive behaviors by nudging users at the right time, not just telling them what to do.

For example:

- Sending movement reminders after extended sedentary periods
- Suggesting a protein-based snack during energy dips
- Highlighting streaks in consistency to reinforce identity-based habits
- Offering "if-this-then-that" logic (e.g., "if you didn't sleep well, consider delaying intense workouts today")

These micro-interventions increase adherence and reduce the chance of dropping off due to life's inevitable curveballs.

6. Long-Term Progress Tracking That Actually Matters

Traditional tracking often obsesses over surface-level metrics: weight, calorie intake, minutes exercised. AI systems take a deeper approach. They look for trends across multiple dimensions — stress, energy, motivation, inflammation, recovery, and metabolic response.

Instead of "Did I lose 5 pounds?" the questions become:

- "Am I sleeping better?"
- "Is my energy more stable during the day?"
- "Has my recovery improved over the past 3 weeks?"
- "Is my stress response better managed?"

These are meaningful indicators of real, sustainable progress — and AI can surface them in ways that build motivation, not shame.

Real-World Example

What Happened
A small digital marketing agency implemented a wellness benefit using an AI-integrated platform. Employees wore health trackers, received daily fitness and nutrition recommendations, and got nudges to adjust based on their unique data (e.g., sleep quality, step count, hydration).

What Went Right
Engagement was high. Absenteeism dropped, mood and focus scores improved, and employees reported feeling supported without pressure. Importantly, many started forming sustainable habits — morning walks, protein-first meals, improved bedtime routines — not because of forced compliance, but because the AI made it easy to stay on track.

What We Learn From It
When AI removes friction and respects individual variation, people don't need motivation — they just need momentum. The right micro-decisions, delivered consistently, produce real change over time.

AI isn't just helping people get fitter or eat better — it's changing the rules entirely. It removes the guesswork, adapts to life's realities, and helps people stay consistent without obsession. It provides not only tools, but *intelligent support* — 24/7, personalized, and judgment-free.

Done right, AI becomes a quiet coach in your pocket — one that always knows what your body needs next.

Next Steps
Now that we've seen how AI creates real, measurable value in fitness and nutrition, it's time to clear the air. In the next section, we'll break down the biggest **Myths About Technology and Health** — and why most fears around AI in wellness are outdated, misunderstood, or flat-out wrong.

Breaking Myths About Technology and Health

The idea of AI helping you train, eat, and recover better still makes some people uneasy. Not because the science isn't sound — but because the assumptions around technology in health are often rooted in fear, hype, or outdated thinking. Misconceptions thrive when change moves faster than public understanding.

This section is about clearing the air. Because if you're making decisions based on myths, you're likely missing out on tools that could unlock dramatic improvements in your health, energy, and long-term resilience.

Let's break down the most common myths — and what the evidence actually shows.

Myth #1: "AI is Cold and Robotic — It Can't Understand the Human Body"

The Reality:
AI doesn't need to "understand emotions" to be effective. It works by identifying patterns in physiological data — far earlier and more accurately than humans can. In fact, AI-based systems are often *more* empathetic in practice because they adjust based on what your body *needs*, not what it's *supposed* to do on paper.

If your recovery is low, it doesn't bark "try harder." It adapts. It backs off. It allows room for grace. That's not robotic — it's intelligent.

In truth, AI is often better at respecting your body than traditional plans ever were.

Myth #2: "AI Replaces Human Coaches and Connection"

The Reality:
AI doesn't replace coaches — it enhances them. It provides real-time insights, so coaches spend less time collecting data and more time focusing on strategy, motivation, and mindset.

For solo users, AI fills the gap when a coach isn't accessible or affordable. It offers 24/7 support, contextual guidance, and habit tracking — far beyond what a human can deliver at scale.

Great health outcomes are built on consistency and feedback. AI delivers both, without judgment or delay.

Myth #3: "Tracking Everything Is Obsessive and Unhealthy"

The Reality:
It's not the *tracking* that's unhealthy — it's the *mindset behind it*. When done manually, tracking can feel tedious and controlling. But AI passively collects and interprets data in the background, freeing you from constant attention.

What you get isn't just numbers — it's meaning. Trends. Adjustments. Encouragement. Not "you failed," but "here's how to pivot."

Used well, AI removes pressure. It supports awareness, not obsession.

Myth #4: "AI Only Works If You're Already Fit or Tech-Savvy"

The Reality:
This is one of the most damaging myths — and flatly untrue.
Today's best AI wellness platforms are built for real people, not elite athletes or engineers.

- If you can wear a ring or a watch, AI can support you.
- If you can log a meal or sync an app, AI can personalize your plan.
- If you can answer a few onboarding questions, AI can detect patterns you'd never spot on your own.

Some of the most profound results come from beginners — because AI meets you *exactly* where you are.

Myth #5: "AI Is Just a Marketing Gimmick"

The Reality:
Plenty of companies throw "AI" into their branding without using true adaptive technology — and that's fair criticism. But the real thing? It's not a buzzword. It's a capability shift.

Genuine AI in wellness uses:

- Machine learning to refine recommendations over time
- Real-time biometric feedback to personalize plans
- Behavioral science to improve habit formation
- Predictive modeling to prevent injury, burnout, or regression

If a platform only spits out cookie-cutter advice, it's not AI — it's a glorified calculator. The key is choosing tools that *learn* from you.

Myth #6: "Technology Disconnects Us From Our Bodies"

The Reality:
Used poorly, any technology can create detachment. But the right AI tools do the opposite — they *strengthen* body awareness by helping you correlate what you feel with what's actually happening inside.

You learn what real recovery feels like. You notice how food timing affects focus. You begin to spot stress patterns before they hit. That's *reconnection*, not detachment.

AI doesn't override your intuition — it trains it.

Real-World Insight

What Happened
A corporate wellness manager was hesitant to roll out wearable tech to their team, worried it would increase pressure, anxiety, or tech fatigue. After a pilot with a small group using an AI-enabled system, the results flipped the narrative.

What Went Right
Employees reported feeling *more* in control, not less. They appreciated the non-judgmental, data-based nudges. Burnout scores decreased. Energy scores rose. Most importantly, participants said they learned more about how their body functioned in six weeks than in years of trial and error.

What We Learn From It
AI isn't about replacing human insight — it's about equipping it. And when used responsibly, it doesn't create dependency. It creates *empowerment*.

Final Takeaway

Fears about AI in health are often based on the worst examples of technology — not the best. The reality is this: done right, AI removes shame, simplifies decision-making, and strengthens personal agency.

It doesn't replace wisdom. It *amplifies it* — quietly, consistently, and at scale.

Next Steps
To see these principles in action, we'll now explore **Case Studies of Early AI Adoption** — from solo users to small teams — and how intelligent systems have already transformed real-world health journeys.

Case Studies of Early AI Adoption

While AI in health and fitness may still sound futuristic to some, it's already delivering tangible results in the real world — not just for athletes or early adopters, but for busy professionals, small teams, and everyday individuals who want sustainable change. These early use cases highlight what's possible when intelligent systems are applied to human wellness with empathy, precision, and practicality.

Each story below illustrates a different context — but all share one core insight: when AI is used to *guide*, not dictate, people make better decisions, recover faster, and stick to their goals longer.

Case Study 1: Solo Transformation — The Burned-Out High Performer

Profile:
Nina, a 39-year-old marketing executive, had tried everything: low-carb diets, marathon training, HIIT classes, intermittent fasting. Despite her effort, she plateaued. She was constantly fatigued, bloated, and sleeping poorly.

AI Integration:
Nina started using a wearable ring and a precision wellness app powered by AI. It tracked her sleep cycles, heart rate variability (HRV), and post-meal glucose responses. The AI recommended shifting her workout intensity based on recovery scores and suggested carb reintroduction on specific days of her hormonal cycle.

Results:
Within two months, Nina reported deeper sleep, better digestion, and more stable energy. She trained less frequently but more effectively. Her body composition improved, and — most importantly — she stopped blaming herself for needing rest.

Lesson Learned:
AI didn't give her more to do. It gave her permission to listen — with data-backed confidence.

Case Study 2: Small Team Wellness — Creative Agency in Crisis Mode

Profile:
A 12-person digital creative firm struggled with high stress, sedentary routines, and frequent sick days. Leadership wanted to support wellness without micromanaging.

AI Integration:
The company implemented a lightweight program pairing wearables

with an AI-powered coaching platform. Each employee received personalized fitness and nutrition nudges based on their unique data (sleep, movement, stress levels). No one was forced to compete or report — privacy and autonomy were respected.

Results:
In three months:

- Sick days dropped by 28%
- 10 of 12 employees improved sleep quality
- Daily step counts increased by an average of 22%
- Mood self-assessments improved across the board

Lesson Learned:
When wellness becomes responsive instead of rigid, engagement goes up — even in teams under pressure.

Case Study 3: Midlife Reboot — From "Too Late" to "Just in Time"

Profile:
Jason, a 52-year-old accountant, believed his best health years were behind him. Weight gain, rising blood pressure, and early signs of insulin resistance convinced him it was "just part of aging."

AI Integration:
He began using a metabolic tracking app synced to his smartwatch. The AI learned his glucose patterns, sleep behavior, and dietary habits, and built him a daily feedback loop: when to move, what to eat first, when to avoid certain foods.

Results:

Within four months:

- Jason lost 18 pounds
- His fasting glucose normalized
- He reported more energy than he had in a decade
- He began walking 8,000–10,000 steps daily without forcing himself

Lesson Learned:

AI didn't just help Jason reverse metrics — it helped rewrite a limiting narrative. He realized it wasn't "too late." He just needed *better tools.*

Case Study 4: Fitness Entrepreneur — Scaling Coaching with AI

Profile:

A personal trainer with 50+ clients was burning out. Creating custom plans, chasing check-ins, and adjusting for illness or injury was becoming unsustainable.

AI Integration:

He adopted an AI-enhanced client management platform that integrated with wearables and food logs. The system provided automated updates to workout intensity, nutrition feedback, and recovery guidance — while flagging when clients needed human touchpoints.

Results:

- Client satisfaction rose due to better personalization
- The trainer saved 12+ hours per week
- Retention increased, and so did referrals

Lesson Learned:

AI doesn't replace a coach — it makes them *more available, more effective, and more scalable.*

Case Study 5: Partnered Progress — A Couple's Wellness Journey

Profile:
Lena and Marco, both in their 40s, had different fitness goals and schedules. Lena wanted to improve her strength; Marco wanted to manage stress and improve sleep.

AI Integration:
They used a shared AI-driven platform that personalized each of their fitness, nutrition, and recovery plans — with occasional synced goals (like walks or meals). The system adjusted automatically as each of their data streams evolved.

Results:

- Lena gained lean mass while maintaining energy for her demanding job
- Marco reduced his resting heart rate and began sleeping consistently through the night
- Their relationship improved as they stopped arguing about "what the plan should be" and trusted their personalized guidance

Lesson Learned:
AI can personalize for individuals — and *align* for partnerships. It removes negotiation and replaces it with shared momentum.

What These Cases Show Us

Across all use cases — solo, team, coach, or couple — a few clear patterns emerge:

☑ AI works best when it *adapts* to daily life, not when it imposes rigid control

☑ Results are strongest when AI is used to simplify decisions, not complicate them

☑ The combination of intelligent feedback and personal responsibility drives real, lasting change

☑ Sustainable health doesn't require obsession — just consistent, *context-aware* action

These aren't theoretical advantages. They're already happening, quietly, across industries, demographics, and goals.

AI is no longer an experiment — it's an accelerant. When applied correctly, it reduces guesswork, improves adherence, and empowers people to take back control of their health.

Next Steps
In the next section, we explore **The Human + AI Partnership in Fitness** — how real results come not from machines or motivation alone, but from the synergy between intelligent systems and human insight.

The Human + AI Partnership in Fitness

For all its power, AI isn't magic — and it's not a replacement for human intuition, experience, or personal values. The most sustainable, empowering approach to fitness and nutrition today isn't a war between man and machine. It's a collaboration. A *partnership*.

In this partnership, AI handles what it does best: crunching data, spotting patterns, and adapting recommendations in real time. Humans handle what *we* do best: applying context, choosing priorities, and staying connected to purpose.

When those two forces work together, something remarkable happens — health becomes both more *scientific* and more *sustainable*.

AI as the Engine, You as the Driver

Think of AI as your vehicle's engine control system. It constantly adjusts fuel, air, and performance to keep the engine running smoothly under different conditions. But it's still *you* behind the wheel.

AI optimizes the vehicle. You decide where you're going.

This distinction matters. You don't surrender agency when you use AI in your health routine — you *enhance it*. You shift from reacting blindly to conditions (burnout, weight gain, inflammation) to proactively steering your fitness with insight and strategy.

AI gives you the map. You still choose the road.

Context Still Wins

Let's say your wearable tells you that your recovery is low, and AI recommends rest. But you *feel* energized and want to lift. Should you ignore the AI?

Not necessarily. But you *contextualize* the advice.

Maybe you slept poorly the past few nights but had a stress release this morning. Maybe you're entering ovulation and naturally feeling more powerful. Maybe this is the only time you have to train this week, and lifting improves your mood. *That's valid.*

AI offers guidance — not orders. The best results come when you understand both what your body is telling you *and* what the data suggests.

Coaches, Enhanced — Not Replaced

If you're a fitness or nutrition coach, AI is not your competition. It's your *infrastructure*. It eliminates the need to track every calorie, check every schedule, or chase every update. Instead, it frees you to focus on strategy, connection, and long-term transformation.

Great coaches will always matter. But great coaches + AI systems? That's next-level. You get consistency and insight without losing the empathy, creativity, or nuance only a human can bring.

And for self-guided individuals, AI is like a coach-in-your-pocket — giving structure without shouting, and feedback without judgment.

When the Partnership Fails

Of course, not all AI systems are built well. And not all users know how to interpret or engage with them. Common partnership breakdowns include:

- **Blind compliance:** Taking every AI suggestion as gospel without self-reflection
- **Data overwhelm:** Getting lost in metrics instead of focusing on behavior
- **Ignoring emotion:** Treating health as mechanical rather than also emotional or social
- **Abandoning accountability:** Expecting the tech to *do* the work rather than *guide* the work

To avoid these traps, the user must stay engaged — curious, reflective, and adaptable. AI is the compass. You still hike the trail.

Tactical Best Practices for the Human + AI Model

- **Use AI as a conversation partner, not a commander**
  Ask *why* it's recommending something. Learn from the logic, then decide for yourself.
- **Match AI insights to your life reality**
  Some days, doing "less" is still a win. If AI says to rest and you walk instead — that's still alignment.
- **Keep a weekly review rhythm**
  Use AI dashboards to spot trends, then reflect on what worked and what didn't. Keep agency at the center.
- **Layer AI with values**
  Let your *why* — not your data — drive consistency. The numbers are tools, not the purpose.

Real-World Insight

What Happened
A 45-year-old gym owner used AI to optimize his nutrition, training, and sleep. At first, he followed every prompt exactly — adjusting meals, skipping lifts on low recovery days, and tweaking macros based on glucose data.

What Went Wrong
After a few months, he felt disconnected. He missed group workouts. He ignored what made him feel fulfilled — community, intensity, spontaneity. The AI was technically "right," but his health outcomes plateaued and his joy declined.

What Shifted
He rebalanced. He started weighing data *against* his values and goals. Sometimes he trained hard despite a low score — but managed recovery better afterward. Sometimes he skipped tracking entirely for a day to stay present with family. He used AI as an advisor, not a dictator.

What We Learn

Technology can optimize the body. But *humans optimize the experience*. And without joy, even perfect metrics mean nothing.

Final Thought

The real revolution isn't AI replacing the health journey — it's AI finally catching up to the complexity of *real life*. It allows plans to bend instead of break. It respects recovery. It supports agency.

But it still needs *you* — your context, your priorities, your decisions.

The best version of fitness isn't automated. It's *augmented* — by insight, not oversight.

Next Steps

With the human + AI foundation in place, we now pivot to **Chapter 2: Understanding the Foundations of Health** — where we break down the biological, behavioral, and environmental pillars that all wellness success is built on. Before we optimize, we need to *understand*. Let's get grounded.

CHAPTER 2

Understanding the Foundations of Health

The Science of Energy Balance (Calories In vs. Calories Out)

No matter how advanced health technology becomes — no matter how smart the AI, how customized the plan, or how optimized the supplements — the foundation of body composition still comes down to one fundamental principle: **energy balance**.

Calories in vs. calories out isn't trendy. It's biology. And whether your goal is fat loss, muscle gain, maintenance, or metabolic recovery, understanding this equation is non-negotiable.

Unfortunately, it's also one of the most misunderstood — and misrepresented — concepts in all of fitness and nutrition. Let's clear that up.

What Energy Balance *Actually* Means

Energy balance refers to the relationship between the calories your body takes in through food and drink, and the calories it expends through basic functions, movement, digestion, and other metabolic processes.

The equation looks simple:

Energy Balance = Calories In – Calories Out

- **Calories In** = All energy consumed through food and beverages
- **Calories Out** =
  - Basal Metabolic Rate (BMR): energy your body uses at rest (around 60–75% of daily expenditure)
  - Thermic Effect of Food (TEF): energy used to digest and process food (about 10%)

- Physical Activity: structured exercise and daily movement
- Non-Exercise Activity Thermogenesis (NEAT): small movements like walking, fidgeting, standing

What Happens in Different Energy States

- **Caloric Deficit**
  If you consume *less* energy than you burn, your body draws on stored energy (fat, muscle, glycogen) to make up the difference. Sustained deficits lead to fat loss — and possibly muscle loss if protein and resistance training aren't adequate.
- **Caloric Surplus**
  If you consume *more* energy than you burn, your body stores the excess — ideally as muscle if you're resistance training, or as fat if you're not. This is required for muscle gain but must be managed carefully.
- **Energy Maintenance**
  If intake and output are matched, your body maintains its current weight. This is the zone for longevity, performance, and stability.

Why It's Not *Just* a Math Equation

Calories in vs. calories out is a *law*, not a strategy. But in practice, the equation isn't static.

Variables that change "calories out" include:

- Sleep quality
- Hormonal state (e.g., thyroid, cortisol, insulin)
- Muscle mass
- Stress levels
- Illness or inflammation
- Aging

And variables that change "calories in" accuracy include:

- Underestimating portion sizes
- Hidden calories in sauces, oils, or snacks
- Misleading food labels
- Water retention or digestive irregularities

This is where **AI can shine** — tracking inputs and outputs more precisely, identifying hidden variables, and helping adjust targets dynamically.

Common Misconceptions

- **"If I'm not losing weight, I must have a slow metabolism."**
  While metabolism can vary, most plateaus come from *inconsistent tracking*, *adaptive thermogenesis*, or *changing activity levels* — not metabolic "damage."
- **"I eat clean, so I should be losing fat."**
  Nutrient quality matters, but fat loss still requires a caloric deficit. Clean foods can still be high in energy.

- **"Exercise burns fat directly."**
  Exercise increases calorie expenditure and can shift the balance — but fat loss still depends on *total daily deficit*, not just the hour you train.
- **"Starvation mode will make me gain weight."**
  Severe, prolonged deficits may *slow metabolism*, but they don't *reverse physics*. You won't gain fat in a true deficit — but you may lose muscle or see hormonal disruption if done recklessly.

Real-World Example

What Happened
A 41-year-old client was eating "perfectly" — organic foods, no sugar, lean proteins — but wasn't losing weight. She was tracking

meals by memory, skipping snacks, and overestimating her calorie burn from workouts.

What Changed
Using a wearable and AI-connected food logging tool, she learned that her post-workout smoothies were 600+ calories, her NEAT was lower on work-from-home days, and her metabolism was downregulated due to low sleep and high stress.

What We Learn From It
Energy balance is subtle — and emotional. AI helped her remove the guilt and focus on the math. By making small, consistent changes, she broke her plateau without overhauling her lifestyle.

Tactical Best Practices

- **Know Your Baseline Needs**
  Use calculators or wearables to estimate your Total Daily Energy Expenditure (TDEE)
- **Track for Awareness, Not Obsession**
  Even 3–5 days of honest logging can reveal where hidden calories (or deficits) live
- **Adjust Intelligently**
  If fat loss stalls, lower calories gradually (5–10%) or increase output — not both at once
- **Prioritize NEAT Over Cardio**
  Increasing daily movement (steps, standing, small tasks) often yields better long-term results than adding intense workouts
- **Support Deficits With Protein and Recovery**
  Muscle loss during fat loss is a real risk. Protect your lean mass with training, protein, and rest

Final Thought

Energy balance isn't the *only* factor in health — but it's the foundation. Without understanding how fuel is used, stored, or depleted in your body, all other strategies are like building on sand.

AI won't change the laws of thermodynamics — but it can help you apply them more accurately, with less stress and more personalization.

Next Steps
Now that we've grounded energy balance, we move into the next critical layer: **Macronutrients — Proteins, Fats, and Carbohydrates.** Because *what* you eat matters just as much as *how much* — and different macros create radically different outcomes in energy, recovery, and body composition.

Macronutrients: Proteins, Fats, Carbohydrates

Once you understand **how much** energy your body needs through the lens of calories, the next logical question becomes: **where should those calories come from?** This is where macronutrients — proteins, fats, and carbohydrates — enter the equation. These are the primary building blocks of your diet, and each plays a distinct, irreplaceable role in how your body performs, recovers, and transforms.

In the age of AI-personalized nutrition, macro distribution has gone from generic ratios to hyper-tailored strategies. But even before applying personalization, it's essential to understand the core science behind each macronutrient — and why balance, not bias, wins in the long run.

The Role of Protein: Repair, Rebuild, and Regulate

What It Does:
Protein is essential for tissue repair, muscle maintenance, immune function, and hormone production. It's made up of amino acids — nine of which are *essential*, meaning your body can't make them on its own.

Why It Matters:

- Supports lean muscle during fat loss
- Aids recovery after training
- Reduces hunger via higher satiety
- Helps regulate blood sugar and metabolism
- Critical for aging well (prevents sarcopenia)

AI Optimization Angle:
Modern platforms can calculate your protein needs dynamically based on training intensity, age, and body composition goals — adjusting for recovery, hormonal phases, or metabolic demand.

Baseline Guidelines:

- Fat loss or general health: 0.8–1g per pound of lean body mass
- Muscle building or high-output training: 1–1.2g per pound of lean body mass
- Older adults: Often benefit from *more*, not less — to offset anabolic resistance

The Role of Fats: Hormones, Brain, and Fuel Buffer

What It Does:
Fats are vital for hormone production, cell membrane integrity, brain function, and absorbing fat-soluble vitamins (A, D, E, K). Dietary fat also helps regulate inflammation and supports mood and satiety.

Why It Matters:

- Supports balanced sex hormone levels (testosterone, estrogen, progesterone)
- Provides a slow-burning fuel source
- Helps prevent energy crashes and cravings
- Protects against overly insulin-driven dietary patterns

Types of Fats:

- **Monounsaturated (MUFA):** olive oil, avocado, nuts
- **Polyunsaturated (PUFA):** fatty fish, flaxseed, chia (includes omega-3s)
- **Saturated (limited but not feared):** dairy, red meat, coconut oil
- **Trans fats (avoid entirely):** industrial processed oils, margarine

AI Optimization Angle:
Advanced platforms can adjust fat intake based on energy needs, inflammation markers, and hormonal cues — especially valuable during menstrual cycles, menopause, or adrenal stress phases.

Baseline Guidelines:

- 20–35% of daily calories from fat is appropriate for most adults
- Prioritize whole-food sources and omega-3-rich options

The Role of Carbohydrates: Energy, Performance, and Recovery

What It Does:
Carbs are the body's preferred fuel source — especially for high-intensity training, brain function, and recovery. They're broken down into glucose and stored as glycogen in the liver and muscles.

Why It Matters:

- Fuels anaerobic and strength training
- Restores muscle glycogen after exercise
- Supports mood and cognitive function
- Helps manage cortisol and thyroid function when timed correctly

Types of Carbs:

- **Complex carbs (preferred):** whole grains, legumes, vegetables
- **Simple carbs (strategic use):** fruits, honey, white rice, juice — useful around workouts
- **Refined carbs (limit):** processed snacks, sugary cereals, soda, pastries

AI Optimization Angle:
AI can optimize carb intake and timing based on your activity levels, insulin response (via glucose monitors), sleep quality, and even time of day (circadian rhythm syncing).

Baseline Guidelines:

- Active individuals may need 2–4g of carbs per pound of body weight
- Low-carb may work for sedentary periods or specific goals, but extreme restriction often backfires for long-term energy and performance

Balancing Your Macros

While "calories in vs. out" determines body weight direction, **macros determine body composition, energy, and performance quality**.

Example:

- A 2,000-calorie diet composed of 40% carbs, 30% protein, 30% fat will feel and perform *very* differently than one made of 60% carbs, 20% protein, 20% fat.

The right balance depends on:

- Activity type and intensity
- Body composition goals (gain vs. cut vs. maintain)

- Hormonal and metabolic needs
- Sleep, stress, and lifestyle demands
- Age and gender
- AI-guided feedback over time

Common Pitfalls

- **Over-Restricting a Macro:**
  Demonizing carbs or fats based on diet trends creates imbalances and long-term issues (e.g., low thyroid, poor recovery, mood swings)
- **Not Prioritizing Protein:**
  Undereating protein is one of the fastest ways to sabotage fat loss or strength gains — especially as we age
- **Chronic Low-Carb Training:**
  Lifting heavy or sprinting while carb-deprived often leads to underperformance, elevated cortisol, and poor recovery
- **Ignoring Context:**
  Your ideal macro split will change — across seasons, stress levels, training phases, and life stages

Real-World Example

What Happened
A 36-year-old project manager was eating "low carb" but struggling with sleep and performance during 5am workouts. Her AI-enabled tracker showed elevated resting heart rate, poor HRV, and disrupted glucose patterns.

What Changed
AI recommended reintroducing slow-digesting carbs at dinner and around training windows. She added sweet potatoes, fruit, and oats.

The Result
Her sleep deepened, recovery improved, and her gym performance rebounded. Her energy stabilized during meetings, and cravings dropped.

Lesson Learned
Macronutrients aren't moral. They're tools. When used with context and intelligence — especially through AI — they unlock higher performance *without* restriction.

Tactical Best Practices

- **Start With Protein**: Anchor every meal with a lean protein source — build around that
- **Choose Whole-Food Fats and Fibrous Carbs**: Prioritize satiety, not just calorie count
- **Time Carbs Strategically**: Use most around training, mental work, or stress peaks
- **Let Your Data Inform Your Split**: Use AI (or honest self-tracking) to adjust macros as your body and goals evolve
- **Don't Obsess Over Ratios**: Focus on *patterns* over time, not perfection each day

Final Thought

Macronutrients are not enemies or trends — they're physiological requirements. Understanding how they work together allows you to fuel your goals without falling into dogma or confusion.

AI platforms can now personalize macros at a level never before possible — adjusting for real-time performance, recovery, and emotional signals. But even the best algorithms rely on foundational understanding. When you combine macro literacy with intelligent tech, the result isn't just improved outcomes — it's long-term nutritional freedom.

Next Steps
Now that we've established the role of macronutrients, we'll move into **Micronutrients and Their Overlooked Role** — because the small things (vitamins, minerals, cofactors) often make the biggest difference in energy, immunity, and long-term vitality.

Micronutrients and Their Overlooked Role

Macronutrients may dominate the conversation in diet culture, but micronutrients are the quiet force behind nearly every process in the human body. Vitamins, minerals, and trace elements don't provide calories, yet they determine whether your body can efficiently use the energy and building blocks you consume.

Think of macronutrients as the bricks and wood in building a house. Micronutrients are the nails, screws, wiring, and plumbing. Without them, the structure may stand — but it won't function properly. And in modern diets, micronutrient deficiencies are far more common than most realize.

What Micronutrients Actually Do

Micronutrients influence critical systems such as:

- **Energy production**: B vitamins help convert carbs, fats, and proteins into usable fuel.
- **Oxygen transport**: Iron supports hemoglobin, allowing red blood cells to deliver oxygen.
- **Bone health**: Vitamin D, calcium, and magnesium build skeletal strength and prevent breakdown.
- **Immune defense**: Zinc, selenium, and vitamin C play direct roles in immune response.
- **Nervous system regulation**: Magnesium, potassium, and sodium govern muscle contraction and nerve signaling.
- **Hormone balance**: Iodine supports thyroid hormones; zinc affects testosterone and estrogen production.

Without adequate micronutrients, even the best-designed macronutrient plan underperforms.

Why Deficiencies Are So Common

Despite living in an era of abundant calories, many people suffer from *hidden hunger*: a lack of essential vitamins and minerals even while eating enough (or too much) food.

Key reasons include:

- **Highly processed diets**: Stripped of vitamins, minerals, and fiber
- **Soil depletion**: Modern farming reduces micronutrient density of produce
- **Restrictive diets**: Cutting entire food groups often removes key micronutrients (e.g., B12 from vegan diets, magnesium from low-carb plans)
- **Stress and illness**: Increase demand for nutrients like magnesium, zinc, and vitamin C
- **Aging**: Reduced absorption efficiency, higher need for certain micronutrients

Overlooked Micronutrients That Matter Most

- **Magnesium**: Supports 300+ enzymatic reactions; crucial for sleep, recovery, and stress regulation. Deficiency is rampant.
- **Vitamin D**: Acts more like a hormone than a vitamin; linked to bone health, immunity, mood, and performance. Many are deficient due to indoor lifestyles.
- **Zinc**: Supports immunity, testosterone, wound healing, and taste perception.
- **Iron**: Essential for oxygen transport. Deficiency common among women and endurance athletes.
- **Potassium**: Balances sodium, supports hydration, regulates muscle and nerve function.
- **Selenium**: Powerful antioxidant; supports thyroid function.
- **B Vitamins**: Critical for energy metabolism; deficiencies mimic fatigue and brain fog.

Real-World Example

What Happened
A 28-year-old recreational runner complained of chronic fatigue, poor recovery, and frequent illness despite a "clean" diet. He was convinced his macros were dialed in.

What Changed
Blood testing revealed iron and vitamin D deficiencies. With supplementation and slight dietary changes (iron-rich foods, vitamin D from fortified sources plus sunlight exposure), his energy rebounded within weeks. His training consistency improved, and his susceptibility to colds decreased.

What We Learn
Macros may fuel the engine, but micronutrients determine if the engine can actually *fire*. Overlooking them keeps performance stuck in neutral.

Common Pitfalls

- **Relying solely on multivitamins**: These can fill gaps, but absorption and bioavailability vary widely.
- **Ignoring symptoms of deficiency**: Fatigue, brittle nails, poor sleep, frequent illness, and mood swings often stem from micronutrient gaps.
- **Excess supplementation**: More isn't always better — fat-soluble vitamins (A, D, E, K) can accumulate to toxic levels.
- **One-size-fits-all nutrition plans**: Micronutrient needs shift with age, stress, and activity.

Tactical Best Practices

- **Eat a diverse, colorful diet**: Each color in fruits and vegetables signals different micronutrients.
- **Prioritize whole foods**: Leafy greens, legumes, nuts, seeds, fatty fish, lean meats, and eggs.

- **Check for deficiencies**: Consider blood work for vitamin D, iron, magnesium, and B12.
- **Use supplements strategically**: To fill proven gaps, not as a substitute for balanced eating.
- **Leverage AI tools**: Some platforms can analyze your intake, flag likely deficiencies, and recommend personalized adjustments.

Final Thought

Micronutrients rarely make headlines, but they're often the difference between *feeling fine* and *thriving*. They power the small processes that add up to performance, resilience, and longevity. Ignoring them is like trying to run high-performance software on a computer missing key system updates — eventually, things slow down or break.

AI-assisted nutrition is helping uncover and correct these hidden gaps more effectively than ever. But the foundation remains timeless: variety, balance, and awareness.

Next Steps
Now that we've covered the essential "invisible nutrients," we'll shift to another often-overlooked pillar: **Hydration and Its Impact on Performance**. Because water balance isn't just about thirst — it's about cognitive clarity, endurance, recovery, and even metabolic efficiency.

Hydration and Its Impact on Performance

Water is the most underrated performance enhancer. We tend to obsess over calories, macros, and supplements, yet something as simple as hydration can make or break both physical and cognitive performance. Even mild dehydration — as little as 1–2% of body weight — can impair focus, reduce endurance, and increase fatigue.

Hydration is not just about quenching thirst. It's about maintaining the delicate balance of fluids and electrolytes that keep every cell in the body functioning. When that balance shifts, everything from energy levels to decision-making suffers.

The Physiology of Hydration

Water makes up about 60% of the human body and plays a central role in:

- **Temperature regulation**: Through sweating and evaporation
- **Nutrient transport**: Moving glucose, amino acids, and oxygen to muscles
- **Joint lubrication**: Protecting mobility and preventing injury
- **Electrolyte balance**: Supporting nerve signaling and muscle contraction
- **Waste removal**: Clearing metabolic byproducts like urea and lactic acid

When hydration drops, the body prioritizes survival functions. Performance and recovery are the first to suffer.

Signs of Underhydration

Often, dehydration isn't dramatic — it's subtle. Early signs include:

- Dry mouth or persistent thirst
- Brain fog or trouble focusing
- Increased resting heart rate
- Unusual fatigue or sluggishness during training
- Dark yellow urine

By the time you feel *very* thirsty, you're already behind.

Hydration and Physical Performance

Even a 2% drop in body water can cause:

- Decreased endurance capacity
- Reduced strength output
- Higher perceived exertion (workouts feel harder than they are)
- Slower recovery between sets and sessions
- Elevated core body temperature

In endurance sports, dehydration can increase time to exhaustion by 10–20%. In strength training, it can reduce power output and increase injury risk.

Electrolytes — sodium, potassium, magnesium, and chloride — are equally critical. Without them, hydration isn't effective. This is why athletes don't just drink plain water; they replenish salts lost in sweat.

Hydration and Cognitive Performance

Hydration doesn't just affect the body — it affects the brain. Research shows dehydration can:

- Reduce short-term memory and concentration
- Increase irritability and stress perception
- Slow reaction time
- Worsen decision-making in complex tasks

For business leaders, knowledge workers, and students, this means hydration directly impacts productivity and focus.

Real-World Example

What Happened
A competitive CrossFit athlete experienced repeated performance crashes during summer training. Despite high protein and carb intake, she felt sluggish and frequently cramped.

What Changed
AI-enabled hydration monitoring (through wearable sensors and sweat analysis patches) revealed she was consistently under-replacing sodium and potassium. By increasing electrolyte intake and tracking fluid loss during sessions, her performance rebounded within weeks.

What We Learn
It wasn't lack of training or nutrition — it was a hydration gap. AI turned guesswork into precision, removing a hidden barrier to performance.

Common Pitfalls

- **Relying on thirst alone**: By the time you're thirsty, you're already dehydrated.
- **Overhydrating with plain water**: Can dilute electrolytes and cause hyponatremia.
- **Ignoring sweat rate differences**: Everyone loses water at different speeds — climate, genetics, and fitness level all play roles.
- **Using sports drinks as a crutch**: Many contain excess sugar without tailored electrolyte ratios.

Tactical Best Practices

- **Start hydrated**: Begin the day with 500–750ml of water before coffee or food.
- **Use the urine check**: Pale yellow = hydrated, dark yellow = underhydrated.
- **Match fluids to sweat loss**: Weigh yourself before and after intense sessions; replace 1.5x the weight lost in fluids.
- **Include electrolytes**: Especially in hot climates, endurance sports, or heavy sweaters.
- **Leverage smart tools**: Some wearables and apps can track hydration status and sweat composition.

Final Thought

Hydration is the foundation layer of performance. You can have the best training plan and diet, but if your cells are running dry, nothing else fires efficiently. It's a low-effort, high-return habit that AI tools can now track and optimize with greater accuracy than ever before.

Next Steps

Now that we've explored hydration, we turn to the **Basics of Exercise Physiology** — understanding how the body produces energy, adapts to stress, and builds resilience. This is the science that makes sense of *why* workouts work — and how AI can help maximize those adaptations.

Basics of Exercise Physiology

At its core, exercise is stress — a carefully applied stimulus that challenges the body to adapt. When you lift a weight, sprint, cycle, or practice yoga, you're not just "burning calories." You're triggering a cascade of physiological responses that remodel tissues, balance hormones, and teach your body to perform at a higher level.

Understanding these basics of **exercise physiology** is key to making sense of why certain workouts feel harder, why progress can stall, and how to train smarter instead of just harder. It also sets the stage for how AI can personalize training by interpreting your body's signals.

The Energy Systems That Power Movement

The human body uses three primary energy systems to fuel activity. Each system has a different capacity and speed for producing ATP (adenosine triphosphate) — the body's energy currency.

1. **ATP–PC System (Phosphagen System)**
   - **Duration:** 0–10 seconds
   - **Fuel:** Stored ATP and creatine phosphate
   - **Use Case:** Short, explosive actions like sprints, heavy lifts, jumps
   - **Limitation:** Depletes quickly; needs minutes to recharge

2. **Glycolytic System (Anaerobic Glycolysis)**
    o **Duration:** 30 seconds to 2 minutes
    o **Fuel:** Glucose or glycogen (carbohydrates)
    o **Use Case:** Intense intervals, circuit training, CrossFit-style workouts
    o **Byproduct:** Lactic acid → contributes to "burn" and fatigue

3. **Oxidative System (Aerobic Metabolism)**
    o **Duration:** 2 minutes and beyond
    o **Fuel:** Carbs and fats (requires oxygen)
    o **Use Case:** Steady-state cardio, endurance sports, daily movement
    o **Limitation:** Slowest system, but most sustainable

Adaptation: Why Training Works

Exercise is essentially controlled damage followed by repair:

1. **Stress (workout)** → muscles break down, cardiovascular system strains, nervous system fires harder.
2. **Recovery (rest, sleep, nutrition)** → body rebuilds stronger, more efficient, and more resilient.
3. **Supercompensation** → performance capacity rises above the starting point.

This cycle explains why *progress happens between workouts, not during them.* Push too little, and there's no stimulus. Push too much without recovery, and you risk overtraining. The sweet spot is in applying the right stress and supporting it with the right recovery.

Key Physiological Adaptations

- **Muscular Adaptation**: Hypertrophy (growth), strength gains, increased endurance capacity
- **Cardiovascular Adaptation**: Larger stroke volume, improved VO_2 max, greater efficiency in oxygen delivery
- **Neurological Adaptation**: Improved motor unit recruitment, faster reaction times, better movement coordination
- **Metabolic Adaptation**: Enhanced ability to store glycogen, increased mitochondrial density, improved fat utilization

These adaptations aren't uniform — they depend on training type, volume, intensity, and recovery.

The Role of Hormones

Exercise doesn't just affect muscles; it impacts your endocrine system:

- **Cortisol** rises acutely during training, but chronic overtraining keeps it elevated.
- **Testosterone and growth hormone** spike with resistance training, aiding repair.
- **Insulin sensitivity** improves with activity, helping glucose control.
- **Endorphins and dopamine** boost mood and motivation.

AI-driven tools can track recovery markers like HRV (heart rate variability), resting heart rate, and sleep quality to suggest when your body is primed for adaptation — and when it's asking for rest.

Real-World Example

What Happened
A 35-year-old recreational lifter plateaued despite training six days per week. He added volume and intensity, convinced "more work" was the answer. Instead, he became chronically fatigued and injured his shoulder.

What Changed
A wearable tracked his HRV and recovery status, showing consistently low scores. With AI-guided programming, he reduced sessions to four days, added aerobic conditioning, and improved recovery. Within eight weeks, he broke through his strength plateau.

What We Learn
Exercise is stress — not just movement. Without understanding and respecting recovery, the stress-response cycle breaks down. Smart training isn't about *more*, it's about *better applied*.

Common Pitfalls

- **Overemphasizing "calorie burn"** instead of long-term adaptation
- **Training harder while ignoring poor recovery signals**
- **Sticking to one modality (e.g., only cardio, only weights)** instead of balancing energy systems
- **Neglecting technique and form** in pursuit of intensity

Tactical Best Practices

- **Match training to your recovery capacity**, not just your motivation level
- **Train all three energy systems** with varied intensity, not just one
- **Log or track workouts** to measure progressive overload — don't guess progress

- **Use biofeedback** (HRV, mood, energy levels) to fine-tune training loads
- **Prioritize consistency over extremes** — long-term adaptation beats short bursts of overexertion

Final Thought

Exercise physiology reminds us that the human body is adaptable, but not limitless. Training creates opportunity; recovery makes progress possible. AI is uniquely positioned to bridge these two — guiding when to push, when to hold back, and how to align effort with outcomes.

Next Steps
Now we move to an often underestimated but *vital* piece of the puzzle: **Sleep and Recovery as Hidden Drivers of Progress.** Because no training or nutrition plan works without the body's ability to recharge, repair, and adapt.

Sleep and Recovery as Hidden Drivers of Progress

Most people think results come from training harder or eating cleaner. But the truth is, progress depends just as much — if not more — on what happens *between* the workouts and meals. Sleep and recovery are the unsung heroes of fitness. They dictate whether your training adapts or backfires, whether your body composition improves or stalls, and whether your energy levels feel limitless or drained.

Neglect them, and you're essentially taxing your system without giving it time to repair. Prioritize them, and everything else — strength, fat loss, focus, mood — gets easier.

The Physiology of Sleep in Performance

Sleep isn't downtime. It's active recovery time where the body performs critical tasks:

- **Muscle repair and growth**: Protein synthesis and release of growth hormone peak during deep sleep.
- **Nervous system reset**: The brain consolidates motor skills and reaction pathways learned during training.
- **Hormonal balance**: Cortisol decreases while testosterone and melatonin rise, creating an optimal environment for repair.
- **Immune defense**: White blood cell activity and inflammatory control strengthen resilience.

Even one night of poor sleep can reduce insulin sensitivity, impair decision-making, and decrease exercise output. Chronic sleep debt magnifies these effects, making fat loss, muscle gain, or performance nearly impossible.

Recovery Beyond Sleep

Recovery is broader than sleep alone. It includes:

- **Nutrition for repair**: Protein and micronutrients aid rebuilding; carbs restore glycogen.
- **Active recovery**: Low-intensity activity (walking, mobility work) increases blood flow and reduces stiffness.
- **Stress management**: Breathwork, meditation, or light stretching reduce nervous system strain.
- **Hydration and electrolytes**: Replacing lost fluids accelerates repair and reduces fatigue.

These practices keep the stress–recovery cycle in balance. Without them, training becomes punishment instead of progress.

How Lack of Recovery Shows Up

When recovery is neglected, the signs aren't subtle:

- Plateaus despite hard training
- Elevated resting heart rate
- Persistent fatigue or irritability
- Poor sleep despite exhaustion
- Declining performance or frequent minor injuries
- Reduced motivation to train

What looks like "laziness" is often systemic fatigue. AI tools are now powerful enough to catch these early through HRV trends, sleep scoring, and readiness indicators.

Real-World Example

What Happened
A 29-year-old competitive cyclist kept pushing through double training sessions, believing volume equaled progress. Within months, he plateaued, developed knee pain, and saw his mood collapse.

What Changed
His AI-driven recovery tracker flagged persistent low HRV and poor deep sleep. By reducing intensity on flagged days, adding structured recovery blocks, and prioritizing bedtime consistency, he returned stronger and injury-free within 12 weeks.

What We Learn
Sleep and recovery aren't optional extras. They are the *currency of adaptation*. Without them, hard work gets wasted.

Common Pitfalls

- **Glorifying hustle**: Treating 5-hour nights and nonstop training as a badge of honor
- **Ignoring signals**: Training hard despite soreness, fatigue, or poor sleep
- **Over-relying on stimulants**: Using caffeine or pre-workouts to mask fatigue instead of fixing it
- **Neglecting routine**: Irregular sleep times prevent quality rest even if hours are sufficient

Tactical Best Practices

- **Aim for 7–9 hours of quality sleep**: Consistency matters more than perfection
- **Create a sleep ritual**: Dim lights, avoid screens, and use cues to signal bedtime
- **Leverage naps strategically**: 20–30 minutes can restore alertness without harming nighttime sleep
- **Listen to recovery data**: HRV, resting heart rate, and sleep trackers can guide intensity decisions
- **Balance stress with recovery practices**: Yoga, walking, or meditation can "top off" the recovery tank

Final Thought

Sleep and recovery aren't weaknesses — they're multipliers. Training and nutrition set the stage, but rest locks in the gains. In the modern era, AI makes it easier to track, respect, and optimize recovery so you can push hard *and* bounce back stronger.

Next Steps
With the foundations of health in place — energy balance, macros, micros, hydration, physiology, and recovery — it's time to get practical. **Chapter 3: Getting Started with AI Tools** will guide you in selecting, setting up, and using AI-driven platforms that bring all of this knowledge to life in a personalized, data-driven way.

CHAPTER 3

Getting Started with AI Tools

Overview of AI Apps for Fitness Tracking

The days of logging workouts in a notebook or manually entering reps into a spreadsheet are fading fast. Today, **AI-powered fitness apps** can track activity, interpret performance, and provide real-time coaching — often with more precision and adaptability than human trainers working alone. But not all tools are equal. To get the most out of them, it's important to understand what they offer, how they differ, and what role they play in your health journey.

What Makes an App "AI-Powered"?

Not every app that claims to use AI truly does. A rule-based program that spits out pre-set workouts isn't artificial intelligence — it's just automation. True AI fitness apps have three defining features:

1. **Adaptive Learning**: They update recommendations based on your performance, recovery, and behavior.
2. **Pattern Recognition**: They spot trends in your data (like declining recovery scores or movement patterns) and act before problems surface.
3. **Personalization at Scale**: They tailor training to *you* specifically, not to a generic "user profile."

Core Capabilities of AI Fitness Apps

- **Workout Generation**: Tailored sessions that adapt daily to your readiness, available equipment, and goals.
- **Form Feedback**: Some apps use motion tracking (via smartphone camera or wearables) to provide real-time technique correction.
- **Progressive Overload Management**: Automatically adjusting sets, reps, or weights as you improve.
- **Recovery Integration**: Syncing with wearables to modify intensity based on sleep, HRV, or fatigue signals.
- **Injury Prevention**: Identifying risk trends (like declining movement quality or overuse patterns) before they escalate.

- **Motivation & Accountability**: Nudges, reminders, and goal reinforcement at times you're most likely to need them.

Popular Types of AI Fitness Tracking Apps

1. **Wearable-Integrated Platforms**
   - Examples: Whoop, Oura, Fitbit Premium
   - Focus: Recovery, readiness scores, activity tracking
   - Strength: Great at monitoring physiology in real time
2. **AI Workout Generators**
   - Examples: Freeletics, Fitbod, Tempo AI
   - Focus: Daily workout creation based on goals and available equipment
   - Strength: Eliminates decision fatigue, adapts over time
3. **Form and Motion Analysis Apps**
   - Examples: Kaia Health, Vi Trainer, Onyx
   - Focus: Using phone camera or sensors to correct exercise form
   - Strength: Safer training without a human coach present
4. **Holistic Platforms**
   - Examples: Ultrahuman, Apple Fitness+, Future
   - Focus: Integration of exercise, recovery, and sometimes nutrition
   - Strength: One-stop-shop experience with broader context

Real-World Example

What Happened
A 34-year-old consultant struggled to stay consistent with strength training while traveling. He often skipped workouts because he lacked equipment or didn't know what to do in a hotel gym.

What Changed
He adopted an AI-powered workout generator that adjusted daily based on his recovery score and available tools (bodyweight, bands,

dumbbells). The app delivered structured 20–30 minute routines that fit his travel lifestyle.

Results

Instead of "all or nothing," he trained consistently 4–5 times per week, even in chaotic schedules. His strength and energy improved steadily without requiring complicated planning.

Lesson Learned

AI doesn't just build better workouts — it removes the barriers to starting. Consistency is easier when the decision-making is automated.

Common Pitfalls

- **Confusing automation with intelligence**: Many apps still rely on static templates disguised as personalization.
- **Overtracking**: Drowning in data without understanding the "so what."
- **Ignoring human context**: No app can know if you had a stressful argument or a draining workday. You must layer judgment on top of insights.
- **Shiny object syndrome**: Switching tools too often prevents meaningful progress tracking.

Tactical Best Practices

- **Choose an app that fits your lifestyle, not just your goals** (e.g., frequent traveler? Pick one with minimal equipment options).
- **Sync your wearables** to give apps richer context on recovery, stress, and activity.
- **Review trends weekly, not daily** to avoid micromanaging every fluctuation.
- **Listen to your body first, AI second** — it's a tool, not a dictator.
- **Commit to one platform for 90 days** before evaluating effectiveness.

Final Thought

AI apps for fitness tracking are powerful not because they replace discipline, but because they simplify it. They take guesswork out of the equation, reduce decision fatigue, and create space for consistency. For many, this is the difference between starting and quitting.

Next Steps
Tracking movement is only half the story. Nutrition drives just as much progress, if not more. In the next section, we explore **AI Diet Planners and Meal Recommendation Engines** — and how they're transforming the way we eat, shop, and sustain healthy habits.

AI Diet Planners and Meal Recommendation Engines

If training sets the stage, nutrition determines how well the performance plays out. Yet for many people, diet is the hardest part of the health equation. Planning meals, balancing macros, tracking portions, and avoiding food fatigue can feel overwhelming. This is exactly where **AI diet planners and meal recommendation engines** shine — not by creating rigid rules, but by simplifying food decisions in a personalized, adaptive way.

What AI Brings to the Table

Traditional diet plans are static: a pre-written meal template that assumes everyone eats the same foods, at the same times, with the same preferences. AI disrupts this by building dynamic, data-driven guidance that evolves with the user.

Key features include:

- **Personalization**: Tailors meals to your caloric needs, macros, allergies, and cultural food preferences.
- **Adaptive Adjustments**: Changes recommendations based on activity level, recovery status, or real-time metrics (e.g., glucose data).
- **Behavioral Nudges**: Suggests practical swaps when cravings or lifestyle challenges arise.
- **Meal Variety Algorithms**: Rotates ingredients and recipes to reduce "food boredom."
- **Integration with Wearables**: Syncs activity and recovery data to adjust meal size or timing dynamically.

Common Use Cases

1. **Macro-Based Precision**
   Apps that align protein, fat, and carb targets with your goals — adjusting daily based on training load.
2. **Glucose-Responsive Eating**
   Platforms synced with continuous glucose monitors (CGMs) recommend foods and timings to stabilize blood sugar.
3. **Time-Saving Meal Prep**
   Automated weekly grocery lists and batch cooking suggestions built around your calendar.
4. **Cultural and Preference Filters**
   AI tools can exclude foods (e.g., vegetarian, halal, kosher, dairy-free) and still provide diverse, satisfying options.
5. **Habit-Building Nutrition**
   Instead of overwhelming calorie tracking, some apps suggest one or two changes at a time — like swapping a sugary breakfast for protein-first meals.

Real-World Example

What Happened
A 42-year-old father of two was stuck in a cycle of takeout lunches and late-night snacking. Despite working out three times a week, he wasn't losing fat and often felt sluggish.

What Changed
He adopted an AI meal planner synced with his wearable. The system recognized his high stress and poor sleep patterns, so it prioritized slow-digesting carbs earlier in the day, protein-rich snacks in the afternoon, and magnesium-containing foods at dinner. It also generated quick lunch recipes he could prep in under 10 minutes.

Results
Within 90 days, he lost 12 pounds, improved afternoon energy, and cut takeout meals by 80%. Importantly, his family started eating healthier alongside him.

What We Learn
AI doesn't just change *what* you eat. It changes how sustainable eating feels by removing friction and decision fatigue.

Common Pitfalls

- **Over-Reliance on Algorithms**: Blindly following recommendations without considering hunger cues or cultural context.
- **Ignoring Quality**: Hitting macros with processed foods is possible — but not optimal for long-term health.
- **Feature Overload**: Some platforms overwhelm users with too many recipes, lists, or metrics.
- **Inconsistent Input**: If meals aren't logged honestly, AI recommendations lose accuracy.

Tactical Best Practices

- **Start Simple**: Use AI for one problem at a time (e.g., lunch planning, macro alignment) instead of overhauling your entire diet.
- **Sync With Other Data**: Wearables and CGMs give meal engines real-time context for better recommendations.
- **Prioritize Whole Foods**: Let the AI guide choices, but bias toward minimally processed ingredients.
- **Review Weekly**: Reflect on how recommendations feel — energy, mood, digestion — not just calories.
- **Use It as a Guide, Not a Dictator**: Combine AI suggestions with your preferences and intuition.

Final Thought

Food is deeply personal — shaped by culture, emotion, and routine. AI doesn't remove that humanity; it enhances it by reducing friction, automating planning, and making healthier eating *easier to sustain*. The real breakthrough is not "perfect diets," but practical, personalized nutrition that adapts as your life changes.

Next Steps
Now that we've looked at how AI can personalize your meals, we'll turn to the hardware side of the equation: **Wearables — Smartwatches, Rings, and Sensors.** These devices collect the data that powers AI insights, making them the backbone of modern health intelligence.

Wearables: Smartwatches, Rings, and Sensors

Wearables have become the front line of the AI health revolution. They sit on your wrist, finger, or skin — quietly collecting streams of data that were once only available in labs or hospitals. From heart rate and sleep cycles to glucose and oxygen saturation, these devices transform your body into a continuous feedback system.

Paired with AI, wearables turn raw data into actionable insights, helping you make smarter decisions about training, nutrition, recovery, and even daily routines.

Categories of Wearables

1. **Smartwatches**
   o **Examples**: Apple Watch, Garmin, Fitbit
   o **Strengths**: Step count, heart rate tracking, GPS, workout detection, notifications
   o **Use Cases**: Everyday wellness, performance tracking, lifestyle integration
   o **AI Advantage**: Combine movement, stress, and recovery data for holistic recommendations
2. **Smart Rings**
   o **Examples**: Oura Ring, Ultrahuman Ring Air, Circular Ring
   o **Strengths**: Sleep quality, HRV, body temperature, recovery readiness
   o **Use Cases**: Subtle, all-day wear without screen distraction
   o **AI Advantage**: Exceptional for recovery monitoring and circadian rhythm insights
3. **Dedicated Sensors**
   o **Examples**: Whoop band, Dexcom (continuous glucose monitor), CORE Temp sensor
   o **Strengths**: Single-metric precision (glucose, lactate, body temp, sweat composition)
   o **Use Cases**: Athletes, medical monitoring, high-performance training
   o **AI Advantage**: High-resolution, real-time feedback for data-driven interventions

The Data They Collect

- **Heart Rate & HRV (Heart Rate Variability)**: Indicators of stress, recovery, and readiness
- **Sleep Staging**: Breakdown of REM, deep, and light sleep cycles
- **Movement & Activity**: Steps, training volume, and non-exercise activity (NEAT)
- **Calories Burned**: Estimated from activity and basal rate
- **Temperature**: Early illness detection, menstrual cycle tracking, and recovery markers
- **Blood Oxygen (SpO$_2$)**: Especially useful for endurance athletes and sleep apnea screening
- **Glucose Monitoring (via CGMs)**: Personalized insights into food response and metabolic health

Real-World Example

What Happened
A 46-year-old consultant felt constantly fatigued despite exercising regularly and eating "well." He wore a smartwatch but ignored the data.

What Changed
Switching to a smart ring integrated with an AI recovery app revealed he was consistently sleeping less than 6 hours and spiking glucose late at night with heavy dinners. With feedback loops in place, he shifted meal timing and bedtime routines.

Results
Within six weeks, his recovery scores rose, his afternoon crashes disappeared, and he finally broke through his fat-loss plateau.

What We Learn
The wearable alone wasn't the solution — it was the **AI interpretation of the data** that turned noise into actionable strategy.

Common Pitfalls

- **Data Overload**: Collecting too many metrics without knowing which ones matter
- **Inaccuracy in Certain Contexts**: Wrist-based heart rate can struggle during strength training
- **Chasing Scores Instead of Listening to the Body**: Recovery score is useful, but not gospel
- **Device Fatigue**: Wearing multiple trackers without integrating them into a single platform

Tactical Best Practices

- **Pick one device that matches your goals**: Smartwatch for all-around, ring for recovery, sensor for precision
- **Sync your wearable with AI platforms**: Data is only useful if it's interpreted
- **Focus on trends, not single-day scores**: Improvement comes from long-term consistency
- **Calibrate data with self-awareness**: Use how you feel alongside what the device reports
- **Review weekly patterns**: Sleep cycles, activity balance, recovery — not just steps or calories burned

Final Thought

Wearables are no longer gimmicks. They're powerful biofeedback systems that bring lab-grade insights into daily life. But the devices themselves aren't the magic — it's the partnership with AI that translates metrics into meaningful actions. With the right wearable and platform, you stop guessing and start aligning your training, nutrition, and recovery with what your body truly needs.

Next Steps

With wearables powering the data stream, the next evolution is coaching. In the following section, we'll compare **AI Workout Coaches vs. Traditional Trainers** — and explore how technology is reshaping the role of human guidance in fitness.

AI Workout Coaches vs. Traditional Trainers

For decades, the gold standard of fitness guidance was hiring a personal trainer — someone to write your program, watch your form, and motivate you to stay consistent. With the rise of AI-driven workout coaches, many now wonder: can a digital coach really replace the human touch?

The reality is more nuanced. AI and traditional trainers each have strengths and limitations. The future of coaching isn't about replacing one with the other — it's about understanding how they differ and where they complement each other.

What AI Coaches Do Well

1. **24/7 Availability**
   AI platforms never sleep. They adapt workouts instantly, whether you're training at 6am, on your lunch break, or in a hotel gym.
2. **Real-Time Adaptation**
   Based on recovery scores, sleep, or performance, AI can automatically scale intensity up or down. No human can adjust this fast across hundreds of data points.
3. **Cost-Effective Personalization**
   AI offers custom programs at a fraction of the price of in-person sessions. For many, this opens access to structured coaching that was previously unaffordable.

4. **Data-Driven Precision**
   AI can integrate inputs from wearables, nutrition trackers, and performance logs — creating a holistic plan that evolves continuously.
5. **Consistency Without Judgment**
   AI coaches don't shame you for missing workouts. They simply recalculate and re-route. This lowers the barrier to restarting after setbacks.

Where Human Trainers Still Excel

1. **Technique Correction in Real Time**
   While some AI apps use cameras for form analysis, nothing replaces in-person feedback for subtle movement patterns and safety.
2. **Motivation and Accountability**
   The emotional connection with a trainer — knowing someone is expecting you — drives adherence beyond what most apps can offer.
3. **Contextual Coaching**
   Trainers factor in your mood, stress from work, or even life events that no wearable can detect.
4. **Creativity and Variety**
   Humans can improvise, change the plan on the fly, and add personal touches to keep workouts engaging.
5. **Relationship and Support**
   For many, the social interaction itself is part of the value. Trainers provide encouragement that AI can't fully replicate.

The Hybrid Future: Human + AI

The strongest model isn't either/or — it's **both**.

- Trainers use AI dashboards to see recovery scores, sleep, and nutrition trends, giving them richer insight into a client's state.

- AI handles repetitive tasks (progress tracking, workout generation, macro adjustments), freeing trainers to focus on higher-value coaching.
- Clients get the best of both worlds: personalized data-driven guidance plus the accountability and empathy of a human.

Example:
A trainer managing 30 clients can't realistically monitor every detail of each client's recovery, sleep, and nutrition. With AI integration, they get alerts when someone's recovery dips or when progress stalls. That allows them to step in with human context at the right time.

Real-World Example

What Happened
A boutique fitness studio integrated AI workout apps with its coaching services. Members received adaptive programs via the app but also had weekly in-person check-ins.

Results

- Attendance increased because members had flexible workout options.
- Trainers spent less time writing programs and more time focusing on form, motivation, and education.
- Members felt supported both in and out of the gym.

What We Learn
AI didn't replace trainers — it *amplified* them. The studio scaled personalization without losing the human connection.

Common Pitfalls

- **Assuming AI is "good enough" for everyone**: Beginners often need real-time form feedback before going digital-only.
- **Trainers fearing replacement**: The best trainers see AI as leverage, not competition.
- **Over-trusting AI metrics**: Numbers don't capture everything — stress, enjoyment, and goals still matter.

Tactical Best Practices

- **For Individuals**: Use AI for structure and flexibility, but seek human feedback periodically.
- **For Trainers**: Integrate AI tools into your service to scale and differentiate, not compete.
- **For Businesses**: Pair digital coaching with human accountability to maximize retention and results.

Final Thought

AI workout coaches offer structure, adaptability, and affordability. Human trainers offer context, creativity, and connection. The smartest path forward is not to choose one but to combine them. Together, they can deliver a level of personalization and accountability that neither could achieve alone.

Next Steps
Now that we've compared AI coaching to human training, we'll explore how to **Integrate Apps for a Unified Experience** — because the real magic happens when your workout tracker, diet planner, and wearable all speak the same language.

Integrating Apps for a Unified Experience

The modern fitness and nutrition landscape is full of powerful tools — wearables, workout apps, diet planners, recovery trackers. But too often, they live in silos. Your smartwatch tracks sleep, your workout app logs sets and reps, your meal planner calculates macros — and none of them "talk" to each other. The result is fragmented data and incomplete insights.

The next frontier in personal health isn't just having great apps. It's about **integration** — building a unified ecosystem where all your tools sync, share, and collaborate to provide one clear picture of your health.

Why Integration Matters

- **Eliminates Blind Spots**: Sleep and recovery data should influence your workout plan. Nutrition intake should reflect training volume. Without integration, these factors remain disconnected.
- **Reduces Decision Fatigue**: Instead of juggling five dashboards, you get one central view.
- **Improves Accuracy**: Combining metrics (e.g., HRV + nutrition + training) allows AI to make smarter, more context-aware recommendations.
- **Supports Long-Term Trends**: Integrated data shows how lifestyle factors interact over months, not just day to day.

How Integration Works

1. **Data Sharing Across Platforms**
   Many apps now connect through APIs (Application Programming Interfaces). For example, Apple Health or Google Fit can act as central hubs where multiple apps deposit data.

2. **AI Aggregators**
   Some platforms (e.g., Ultrahuman, Whoop integrations, TrainingPeaks) act as "brains," pulling inputs from wearables, nutrition trackers, and training logs, then translating them into cohesive recommendations.
3. **Smart Automation**
   Integrations can trigger actions. Example: poor sleep detected → diet app adjusts carb timing → workout app reduces session intensity.

Real-World Example

What Happened
A 37-year-old tech executive used a smartwatch, a calorie-tracking app, and a fitness program separately. Each gave useful data, but none explained why he was constantly tired.

What Changed
By syncing all three into a single AI hub, he discovered the pattern: his poor sleep was spiking cortisol, which increased late-night snacking. The diet app adjusted macros, the workout app cut intensity on poor recovery days, and the AI recommended earlier wind-down routines.

Results
Energy stabilized, fat loss accelerated, and training felt sustainable instead of draining.

What We Learn
The breakthrough wasn't adding another tool — it was connecting the ones he already had.

Common Pitfalls

- **App Overload**: Too many tools without integration leads to confusion and drop-off.
- **Partial Syncing**: Not all apps share full data sets; sometimes only surface-level metrics get synced.
- **Ignoring User Experience**: Even if data is synced, clunky interfaces discourage use.
- **Privacy Oversight**: Integration means more data sharing — users must be mindful of what information is stored and where.

Tactical Best Practices

- **Pick a Central Hub**: Apple Health, Google Fit, or another aggregator should be your "single source of truth."
- **Audit Your Tools**: Choose 2–3 apps that integrate well instead of juggling 6+ with no connection.
- **Prioritize Actionable Data**: Integration should drive decisions (e.g., adjust training), not just consolidate numbers.
- **Check Privacy Settings**: Make sure data-sharing agreements align with your comfort level.
- **Review Weekly Summaries**: Use unified dashboards to spot trends, not to micromanage every data point.

Final Thought

Integration is the difference between collecting information and creating intelligence. By unifying apps and wearables into one ecosystem, you remove noise, reduce decision fatigue, and empower AI to provide clear, actionable guidance. The future isn't more apps — it's smarter ecosystems.

Next Steps

Now that we've explored integration, the next step is personalization. In the following section, we'll look at **Choosing the Right Tool for Your Personal Goals** — helping you filter the growing marketplace of AI tools to find the ones that fit your lifestyle, preferences, and objectives.

Choosing the Right Tool for Your Personal Goals

With so many apps, wearables, and AI-driven platforms available, it's easy to feel overwhelmed. The danger is adopting the "shiniest" tool instead of the *right* tool. The truth is, no single app or device works for everyone. The best choice depends on your specific goals, lifestyle, and even personality.

Choosing wisely is critical — because the wrong tool doesn't just waste money. It can also create friction, frustration, and ultimately derail your consistency.

Step 1: Define Your Primary Goal

Ask yourself: *What outcome matters most right now?*

- **Fat Loss** → Prioritize calorie/macro tracking apps and behavior-change nudges.
- **Muscle Gain** → Use platforms that emphasize progressive overload and recovery tracking.
- **Endurance** → Focus on wearables and apps with strong heart-rate and VO$_2$ max analytics.
- **Stress Management & Longevity** → Choose tools centered on sleep, recovery, and HRV.
- **General Wellness** → Look for all-in-one platforms with balanced nutrition, movement, and recovery guidance.

Step 2: Match the Tool to Your Lifestyle

The best tool is the one you'll actually use. Consider:

- **Do you prefer simplicity?** → A smart ring with a single daily readiness score may be better than a data-heavy smartwatch.
- **Do you travel frequently?** → Look for mobile-friendly apps with bodyweight or minimal-equipment options.
- **Are you motivated by numbers?** → Choose apps with detailed analytics and progress tracking.
- **Do you crave accountability?** → Hybrid platforms with human coaching elements may serve you better than fully automated AI.

Step 3: Evaluate Integration Potential

Your chosen tool should "play well with others." A great workout app loses value if it can't sync with your wearable or nutrition tracker. Always check:

- Can it connect to Apple Health, Google Fit, or your main wearable?
- Does it export/import full data or just basic metrics?
- Does it fit into a broader ecosystem you're already using?

Step 4: Consider Personality Fit

- **Data-Driven Users**: Thrive on detailed dashboards and real-time adjustments.
- **Minimalists**: Prefer single-score outputs (e.g., a readiness rating) without overwhelm.
- **Gamers/Competitors**: Do well with platforms that use streaks, leaderboards, or badges.
- **Independent Learners**: Appreciate educational layers that explain the "why" behind recommendations.

Real-World Example

What Happened
A 31-year-old project manager wanted to lose weight but kept abandoning complex tracking apps. She hated logging every bite.

What Changed
She switched to an AI diet app that focused on "nudges" and simple swaps instead of calorie micromanagement. The app integrated with her smartwatch to estimate intake/expenditure balance.

Results
By simplifying the process, she stuck with it long-term, losing 15 pounds and maintaining the habit without food logging burnout.

What We Learn
The best tool isn't always the most advanced — it's the one that matches *your personality and lifestyle.*

Common Pitfalls

- **Chasing Trends**: Buying the latest gadget without a clear purpose.
- **Tool Overload**: Using five apps at once and becoming paralyzed by too much data.
- **Ignoring Sustainability**: Picking tools that are too complex or demanding for your lifestyle.
- **Assuming Expensive = Better**: Price doesn't equal fit. Sometimes a simple wearable outperforms a costly, overengineered one.

Tactical Best Practices

- **Start with your biggest challenge**: Is it food, workouts, or recovery? Choose a tool for that first.
- **Audit every 90 days**: Ask if the tool is still serving you. If not, adjust.

- **Seek integration-ready tools**: Avoid isolated platforms that create data silos.
- **Focus on behavior, not just metrics**: Pick tools that help you *act*, not just measure.
- **Remember your "why"**: Every tool should align with your deeper goal — not distract from it.

Final Thought

Choosing the right AI fitness or nutrition tool isn't about chasing the most advanced technology. It's about aligning the tool with your goals, lifestyle, and preferences. The right choice feels natural, reduces friction, and makes healthy habits easier to sustain.

Next Steps
With tools selected, we now turn to the real magic: **Chapter 4 – Personalization Through Data.** This is where your chosen apps and wearables stop being generic trackers and start creating a deeply customized roadmap built around *your unique body and behavior.*

CHAPTER 4

Personalization Through Data

Gathering Baseline Health Metrics

Before AI can personalize your fitness and nutrition journey, it needs a starting point — a **baseline**. Just like a doctor wouldn't prescribe treatment without first running tests, your AI tools can't make intelligent recommendations without initial data about your body and habits.

Think of this as your *health fingerprint*: a collection of numbers and patterns that describe where you are today. With a clear baseline, AI systems can measure change, identify trends, and adjust your plan in real time. Without it, even the smartest tools are just guessing.

Why Baselines Matter

- **Context for Progress**: Without a starting point, you can't measure improvement.
- **Personalization**: AI needs to know *your* body, not just averages.
- **Risk Management**: Baseline markers can reveal underlying issues (e.g., sleep debt, elevated resting heart rate) before training intensifies.
- **Motivation**: Tangible data makes progress visible — reinforcing small wins.

Key Metrics to Collect

1. **Body Composition & Weight**
   - Weight alone is incomplete; pair it with body fat percentage and lean mass if possible.
   - Tools: smart scales, DEXA scans, calipers, or AI-enabled imaging apps.

2. **Cardiovascular Markers**
   - Resting heart rate (RHR): lower typically = better conditioning.
   - Heart rate variability (HRV): indicates stress and recovery readiness.
   - Blood pressure: vital for long-term health monitoring.
3. **Metabolic Indicators**
   - Basal metabolic rate (BMR) estimates daily energy needs.
   - Blood glucose trends (if using CGMs).
   - Energy levels and hunger patterns (subjective logs).
4. **Sleep & Recovery**
   - Average hours, sleep stages, and consistency.
   - Resting body temperature shifts (especially for hormonal tracking).
5. **Activity & Fitness Level**
   - Daily steps, activity minutes, workout history.
   - VO$_2$ max estimates (common on wearables).
   - Strength benchmarks (basic lifts, push-ups, planks).
6. **Lifestyle Inputs**
   - Stress levels, work schedule, travel habits, nutrition patterns.
   - These may be subjective but are critical for context.

Tools for Collecting Baselines

- **Wearables**: Smartwatches, rings, and bands capture HR, HRV, sleep, steps, and activity.
- **Smart Scales**: Track body weight, fat %, and sometimes muscle/bone mass.
- **Fitness Tests**: Simple push-up, squat, or walking tests establish strength/endurance baselines.
- **Lab Tests (Optional)**: Bloodwork for glucose, cholesterol, vitamin D, etc. for deeper insight.
- **AI Apps**: Some platforms compile all these metrics into one baseline readiness score.

Real-World Example

What Happened
A 38-year-old entrepreneur wanted to "get in shape" but felt lost. He downloaded a fitness app but skipped the baseline setup. The AI delivered random workouts, leaving him sore and discouraged.

What Changed
When he finally completed the baseline metrics (weight, activity history, sleep logs, RHR), the app recalibrated. It cut initial intensity by 30% and focused on recovery first.

Results
He stuck with the program, improved sleep, and regained energy. Progress accelerated — not from doing *more*, but from starting with the right baseline.

What We Learn
Skipping baseline setup creates mismatched recommendations. The better the starting data, the smarter the AI response.

Common Pitfalls

- **Obsessing Over Perfection**: A baseline doesn't need lab precision — trends matter more than exact numbers.
- **Faking Inputs**: Entering "ideal" answers only hurts personalization. Be honest.
- **Collecting But Not Using Data**: Baselines are only useful if integrated into AI platforms.
- **Overloading Metrics**: Focus on a handful of meaningful indicators instead of drowning in numbers.

Tactical Best Practices

- **Record at least one body metric, one cardiovascular metric, and one recovery metric** as a starting point.
- **Use the same tools consistently** (e.g., weigh-in at the same time of day).
- **Repeat every 4–6 weeks** to track trends without obsessing daily.
- **Let AI fill gaps** — if you can't get advanced tests, wearables can provide enough approximation to start.
- **Pair objective data with subjective notes** (energy, mood, hunger) for a fuller picture.

Final Thought

Gathering baseline health metrics is like building a map. Without a clear "You Are Here," the smartest navigation system can't guide you. Baselines give AI the foundation to personalize intelligently, adjust dynamically, and measure progress meaningfully.

Next Steps
With your baselines established, the next step is sharpening the picture of your body itself. In the following section, we'll explore **Using AI for Body Composition Analysis** — and how technology is moving beyond scales to deliver accurate, real-time insight into fat, muscle, and metabolic health.

Using AI for Body Composition Analysis

Step on a traditional scale and you'll see one number: your weight. But that number alone tells a very incomplete story. Two people can weigh the same yet look, feel, and perform dramatically differently based on their body composition — the ratio of fat, muscle, bone, and water in the body.

This is where AI is reshaping the way we measure and understand progress. Instead of relying on static numbers or inaccurate guesses, AI-powered tools now provide more precise, adaptive, and actionable analysis of body composition.

Why Body Composition Matters More Than Weight

- **Performance**: More lean muscle = higher strength and endurance potential.
- **Metabolism**: Muscle tissue burns more calories at rest than fat tissue.
- **Longevity**: Low muscle mass (sarcopenia) is strongly linked to frailty and disease risk with age.
- **Health Risks**: Visceral fat around organs increases risk of diabetes, cardiovascular disease, and inflammation — even if overall weight looks "normal."

Put simply: *it's not about losing weight, it's about losing fat and preserving (or gaining) muscle.*

Traditional vs. AI-Enhanced Methods

1. **Traditional Approaches**
   - **BMI (Body Mass Index)**: Quick but misleading; doesn't distinguish fat from muscle.
   - **Skinfold Calipers**: Operator-dependent and inconsistent.
   - **Bioelectrical Impedance Scales (BIA)**: Widely available but prone to hydration-related inaccuracies.
   - **DEXA Scans & BodPods**: Accurate, but costly and impractical for frequent use.
2. **AI-Enhanced Approaches**
   - **Smart Scales with AI Algorithms**: Use multi-frequency impedance combined with AI to adjust for hydration, age, and body type.
   - **Computer Vision Analysis**: Apps analyze photos or 3D body scans to estimate fat distribution and muscle changes over time.

- o **Predictive Modeling**: AI combines wearable data (HRV, activity, calorie expenditure) with periodic inputs (photos, weight) to create dynamic body comp trends.

How AI Improves Accuracy and Actionability

- **Pattern Recognition**: AI learns from repeated inputs, filtering out day-to-day noise like water retention or digestion.
- **Contextual Adjustments**: It accounts for lifestyle, hydration, and training load instead of treating all data equally.
- **Visualization**: 3D scans and photo tracking show *where* fat is being lost or muscle gained — more motivating than a single number.
- **Integration**: Body comp changes feed into nutrition and workout apps, automatically adjusting macros or training volume.

Real-World Example

What Happened
A 33-year-old office worker grew frustrated when the scale barely moved despite months of strength training. She was convinced her program "wasn't working."

What Changed
Her trainer introduced an AI body composition tool that combined smart scale data with photo-based analysis. The AI revealed she had lost 5 pounds of fat *and* gained 4 pounds of muscle.

Results
Her body fat percentage dropped significantly, her strength improved, and she finally saw visible definition.

What We Learn
Weight alone masked progress. AI-driven body comp analysis told the real story, keeping motivation high.

Common Pitfalls

- **Relying on One Measurement Alone**: No tool is perfect. Single readings (even with AI) can mislead.
- **Short-Term Obsession**: Small fluctuations are normal; long-term trends matter most.
- **Ignoring Lifestyle Data**: Hydration, stress, and sleep can affect readings if not contextualized.
- **Overcomplicating**: More data isn't always better. Focus on 2–3 key trends.

Tactical Best Practices

- **Use Multiple Inputs**: Combine scale readings with photos, performance metrics, and how clothes fit.
- **Track Trends, Not Days**: Review changes weekly or monthly, not daily fluctuations.
- **Sync With Nutrition & Training Apps**: Let AI adjust your plan based on actual body comp changes.
- **Stay Consistent in Conditions**: Weigh or scan at the same time of day, under similar hydration/meal states.
- **Use Visual Feedback**: 3D scans or photo comparisons often motivate more than numbers.

Final Thought

Body composition analysis is moving beyond clipboards and static scales. AI offers a dynamic, contextual view that recognizes the complexity of human bodies. It's not just about accuracy — it's about *actionable insight*. By focusing on fat, muscle, and distribution, AI helps ensure your journey is about true health improvements, not misleading scale numbers.

Next Steps

With body composition covered, we now turn to a fast-growing frontier: **Continuous Glucose Monitoring and AI Insights.** This technology is unlocking real-time understanding of how your body responds to food — and how personalized adjustments can stabilize energy, performance, and long-term health.

Continuous Glucose Monitoring and AI Insights

Blood sugar control is one of the most powerful yet misunderstood levers for health, performance, and longevity. While most people associate glucose tracking with diabetes, continuous glucose monitoring (CGM) has emerged as a powerful tool for anyone who wants to understand how their body responds to food, stress, and exercise.

By pairing CGM sensors with AI-driven platforms, individuals can now see — in real time — how lifestyle choices impact blood sugar and, by extension, energy, mood, and fat storage. This level of visibility was once impossible without frequent finger-prick tests. Today, it's as simple as wearing a small patch on the arm or abdomen.

Why Glucose Matters for Everyone

- **Energy Levels**: Stable glucose equals steady energy; spikes and crashes drive fatigue and cravings.
- **Performance**: Fueling correctly around workouts depends on how your body processes carbs.
- **Metabolic Health**: Chronic spikes increase insulin resistance risk, a precursor to diabetes.
- **Fat Storage**: Frequent surges promote fat storage and make fat loss more difficult.
- **Brain Function**: Glucose instability is tied to mood swings, brain fog, and poor focus.

Even non-diabetics benefit from understanding their "glycemic fingerprint" — the unique way their body reacts to different foods and behaviors.

How CGMs Work

- A small sensor is inserted just under the skin, typically on the arm.
- It measures interstitial glucose (the glucose between cells), not just blood glucose.
- Data streams to a smartphone app in real time.
- AI algorithms interpret the patterns, score meals, and suggest interventions.

AI's Role in Glucose Insights

CGM alone provides raw data. AI makes it actionable:

- **Meal Scoring**: Evaluates how specific foods or combinations affect glucose.
- **Pattern Recognition**: Detects recurring spikes tied to certain meals, stress, or poor sleep.
- **Behavioral Suggestions**: Recommends simple adjustments (e.g., walking after a carb-heavy meal, eating protein first).
- **Predictive Modeling**: Anticipates how future food choices may impact glucose stability.
- **Personalization**: Recognizes that two people may respond very differently to the same food.

Real-World Example

What Happened
Two coworkers wore CGMs and both ate identical oatmeal breakfasts. One experienced a stable glucose response; the other spiked dramatically and then crashed within two hours.

What Changed
The AI platform recommended the second person add protein and fat (Greek yogurt and nuts) to stabilize the meal. It also suggested walking for 10 minutes afterward.

Results
Her glucose curve flattened, energy improved, and mid-morning cravings disappeared.

What We Learn
Nutrition is not "one size fits all." AI-driven CGM feedback personalizes food choices to your biology, not just generic advice.

Common Pitfalls

- **Chasing Perfection**: Not every spike is bad; context matters (e.g., post-workout glucose rise is normal).
- **Overreacting to Data**: Stressing over every fluctuation can cause more harm than good.
- **Short-Term Obsession**: CGMs are most valuable when used for weeks or months to establish patterns, not micromanaged minute by minute.
- **Ignoring Lifestyle Factors**: Sleep, stress, and exercise impact glucose as much as food does.

Tactical Best Practices

- **Test "go-to" meals**: Use CGM + AI feedback to refine your regular diet, not every single food.
- **Pair carbs with protein or fiber**: Reduces glucose spikes and improves satiety.
- **Time carbs around activity**: Workouts increase glucose utilization and reduce spikes.
- **Log sleep and stress alongside meals**: AI can then connect hidden variables to your glucose trends.
- **Use it as a learning tool**: A few weeks of CGM can build long-term nutritional wisdom.

Final Thought

Continuous glucose monitoring is one of the clearest examples of how AI can transform raw health data into personalized action. Instead of generic diet rules, you learn how *your* body responds — giving you control over energy, cravings, and long-term metabolic health.

Next Steps
We've seen how CGMs and AI uncover hidden responses to food. Next, we'll explore **AI-Driven Food Recognition and Logging** — the next leap forward in simplifying nutrition tracking by removing the hassle of manual entry altogether.

AI-Driven Food Recognition and Logging

Ask anyone what the hardest part of getting fit is, and you'll often hear the same answer: **tracking food.** Logging meals can feel tedious, inaccurate, and unsustainable. Most people give up after a few days, which means their nutrition strategy falls apart long before they see real results.

This is exactly where AI-driven food recognition and logging is changing the game. By combining image recognition, barcode scanning, and natural language processing, these tools drastically reduce the friction of food tracking. Instead of manually searching for "chicken breast, grilled, 5 oz," you simply snap a photo or describe your meal — and the AI does the heavy lifting.

How It Works

- **Image Recognition**: Take a photo of your meal. AI identifies foods, estimates portion sizes, and assigns macros/calories.
- **Barcode & Label Scanning**: For packaged foods, scanning a label instantly uploads nutrition data.

- **Voice & Text Logging**: Dictate or type a description ("oatmeal with banana and peanut butter") and AI parses it into measurable values.
- **Pattern Learning**: Over time, the app remembers your frequent meals and creates shortcuts for instant logging.
- **Integration with Wearables**: AI adjusts recommendations dynamically based on activity, recovery, or glucose responses.

Why This Matters

- **Accuracy Without Burden**: Reduces human error and guesswork in portion sizing.
- **Behavioral Sustainability**: People are more likely to track consistently when it takes seconds, not minutes.
- **Personalized Adjustments**: AI can flag nutrient gaps ("low protein at breakfast") and suggest fixes.
- **Immediate Feedback**: Helps users understand how food choices align with their daily goals in real time.

Real-World Example

What Happened
A 29-year-old teacher had failed multiple times with calorie-tracking apps. She found them too time-consuming and stopped after two weeks.

What Changed
She switched to an AI food logging app with photo recognition. Logging meals took less than 10 seconds. The AI flagged she was consistently low in protein and suggested simple additions like Greek yogurt or eggs.

Results
She maintained the habit for 6 months, lost 15 pounds, and reported feeling more in control without food tracking dominating her day.

What We Learn
Ease of use drives adherence. The best nutrition plan isn't the most advanced — it's the one you'll stick with.

Common Pitfalls

- **Portion Estimation Errors**: AI is improving, but large or mixed dishes (e.g., casseroles) may still confuse algorithms.
- **Over-Tracking Mindset**: Some users may become overly focused on numbers instead of overall patterns.
- **Database Gaps**: Ethnic or homemade meals may lack exact matches, requiring approximations.
- **Privacy Concerns**: Photos of meals may raise data security issues; choose reputable platforms.

Tactical Best Practices

- **Combine photo + weight**: For higher accuracy, weigh key items (like protein portions) while AI logs the rest.
- **Focus on consistency, not perfection**: Use logging to see patterns, not to achieve 100% accuracy.
- **Leverage reminders**: Many apps nudge you if a meal isn't logged within a timeframe.
- **Review weekly summaries**: Focus on big trends (protein intake, calorie averages) instead of micromanaging daily.
- **Sync with fitness goals**: Let the app adjust macros dynamically when training volume increases.

Final Thought

AI-driven food recognition is removing the #1 barrier to sustainable nutrition tracking: complexity. By making logging fast, simple, and adaptive, these tools help people stay consistent long enough to see results — without turning every meal into a math exercise.

Next Steps

With food logging simplified, the next frontier is training load. In the following section, we'll dive into **Smart Wearables for Exercise Load Monitoring** — and how AI uses heart rate, motion, and recovery data to balance intensity, prevent overtraining, and optimize performance.

Smart Wearables for Exercise Load Monitoring

One of the most powerful contributions AI has made to fitness is shifting the focus from "how much you worked out" to "how much your body can handle." Traditional tracking used to stop at counting reps, steps, or calories burned. But with **smart wearables** paired with AI, athletes and everyday users alike can now measure *exercise load* — the real physiological stress of a workout — and adapt training accordingly.

What Is Exercise Load?

Exercise load represents the total stress placed on your body during activity. It's not just the number of sets or miles, but the internal effort required to perform them. Two people may do the same workout, but their load can differ dramatically based on conditioning, recovery, and physiology.

Key factors that define load include:

- **Heart Rate & HRV Trends**: Measure how much strain the workout places on cardiovascular and nervous systems.
- **Repetition/Volume Tracking**: Monitors sets, reps, tonnage lifted, or steps taken.
- **Training Intensity Distribution**: Balances easy, moderate, and hard sessions.
- **Recovery Markers**: Links post-exercise recovery needs with actual performance.

How Smart Wearables Track Load

Modern wearables (Whoop, Oura, Garmin, Polar, Apple Watch) do far more than count steps. They measure:

- **Session RPE (Rate of Perceived Exertion)** combined with heart-rate data to estimate training strain.
- **Acute vs. Chronic Load Ratios**: AI compares short-term spikes to long-term capacity, flagging injury risks.
- **Movement Quality**: Some sensors detect form breakdown and asymmetry in lifts or runs.
- **Adaptive Training Zones**: AI recalibrates heart-rate or power zones as your fitness improves.

Why Exercise Load Monitoring Matters

- **Prevents Overtraining**: Ensures you're not stacking high-intensity sessions back-to-back without recovery.
- **Optimizes Progression**: Guides when to increase volume or intensity safely.
- **Reduces Injury Risk**: Early detection of load spikes prevents stress-related breakdowns.
- **Improves Longevity**: Builds resilience by balancing stress and adaptation cycles.

Real-World Example

What Happened
A 27-year-old marathon trainee ran 6 days per week at high intensity, convinced more mileage meant better results. By week 10, she developed knee pain and exhaustion.

What Changed
Her Garmin watch flagged dangerously high acute training load compared to her chronic baseline. The AI-driven app adjusted her plan, replacing two runs with cross-training and recovery work.

Results
She recovered, finished her marathon pain-free, and learned to balance training stress with recovery.

What We Learn
Tracking load, not just mileage or calories, protects performance while sustaining progress.

Common Pitfalls

- **Chasing High Scores**: Some users see load metrics as a competition, ignoring recovery.
- **Ignoring Subjective Feedback**: Numbers don't always capture how you *feel* — soreness, motivation, and stress still matter.
- **Device Accuracy Limits**: Sensors can misread under certain conditions (e.g., wrist HR during lifting).
- **Data Without Action**: Tracking load is only useful if training is adjusted in response.

Tactical Best Practices

- **Track Both Internal and External Load**: Use wearables for HR/HRV plus volume metrics (weight lifted, distance, reps).
- **Look for Trends, Not One-Offs**: Focus on weekly and monthly patterns.
- **Sync With Recovery Data**: Integrate sleep, HRV, and readiness scores to refine intensity planning.
- **Apply the 80/20 Rule**: Keep ~80% of training in lower zones, 20% in high-intensity — AI can help balance this.
- **Review Weekly Summaries**: Use AI dashboards to adjust next week's volume before problems arise.

Final Thought

Smart wearables transform training from guesswork into precision. Instead of pushing harder blindly, you can balance load and recovery in a way that maximizes results and minimizes risk. AI doesn't just track your workouts — it teaches you when to push, when to pause, and how to progress intelligently.

Next Steps
With all this powerful tracking comes a critical question: who controls your data? In the next section, we'll explore **Privacy and Data Protection in Health Tracking** — ensuring that the information guiding your health isn't being misused.

Privacy and Data Protection in Health Tracking

As AI-driven health tools become more powerful, the data they collect also becomes more sensitive. Sleep cycles, heart rate variability, glucose responses, menstrual cycles, stress levels — this isn't just fitness trivia. It's intimate health information that, if misused, could affect insurance eligibility, employment, or even personal security.

While AI can unlock incredible personalization, the flip side is that your health data becomes a valuable commodity. Protecting that data is just as important as tracking it.

Why Health Data Is So Sensitive

- **Identity & Privacy Risks**: Unlike a password, your biometric markers (like heart rate patterns or glucose data) can't be "reset."
- **Insurance & Employment Concerns**: Data leaks could lead to discrimination based on health risks or lifestyle habits.
- **Behavioral Insights**: Sleep or stress tracking can reveal patterns about work hours, habits, and even location.

- **Commercial Exploitation**: Some platforms sell anonymized data to advertisers or pharmaceutical companies.

How Leading Platforms Handle Data

Reputable apps and wearables increasingly emphasize:

- **End-to-End Encryption**: Protects your data from being intercepted.
- **Anonymization**: Removes personal identifiers before data is analyzed or shared.
- **User Consent**: Requires opt-in before data is sold or used for research.
- **Data Portability**: Allows you to download or delete your records.

Still, practices vary. Always review the privacy policy — not the marketing claims.

Real-World Example

What Happened
A major fitness platform faced backlash after reports revealed its "community heatmap" accidentally exposed sensitive military base locations. Soldiers wearing fitness trackers unintentionally revealed patrol routes and base layouts.

What We Learn
Even anonymized data can create real-world risks if not handled carefully. Transparency and safeguards must be non-negotiable.

Common Pitfalls

- **Not Reading Terms of Service**: Many users unknowingly consent to data sharing.
- **Linking Accounts Blindly**: Connecting apps and wearables without checking what data flows where.

- **Assuming All Platforms Are Equal**: Privacy protections vary drastically between companies.
- **Neglecting Account Security**: Weak passwords or no 2FA leave health accounts vulnerable.

Tactical Best Practices

- **Check Privacy Policies**: Look for clear statements on data storage, sharing, and deletion.
- **Use Platforms With Strong Encryption**: End-to-end security is a baseline requirement.
- **Enable Two-Factor Authentication (2FA)**: Protects against unauthorized access.
- **Control Data Sharing**: Only sync apps you trust and actually need.
- **Review and Delete Old Data**: Periodically clean up unused accounts or platforms.

Final Thought

AI-driven health tools are only as trustworthy as the companies that handle your data. The personalization benefits are enormous, but they come with responsibility: to protect your information, demand transparency, and use only platforms that align with your privacy values.

Next Steps
With security and trust established, we now move to **Chapter 5 – AI for Smarter Diet Planning**, where we'll explore how artificial intelligence is transforming nutrition from generic "meal plans" into personalized, adaptive systems that evolve with your body and lifestyle.

CHAPTER 5

AI for Smarter Diet Planning

Customized Meal Plans Using AI Nutrition Engines

Meal planning has always been a stumbling block for people pursuing health goals. Even with the best intentions, many find themselves overwhelmed by questions: *What should I eat? How much protein is enough? How do I balance variety with convenience?* Traditional meal plans tend to be rigid, generic, and unsustainable — they don't adapt when life changes.

AI nutrition engines are rewriting this story. By analyzing your personal metrics, preferences, and lifestyle patterns, these systems generate **dynamic, customized meal plans** that evolve with you. Instead of handing you a static "30-day plan," they act as an intelligent guide that adjusts day to day.

How AI Builds Personalized Meal Plans

- **Baseline Inputs**: Age, weight, activity level, body composition, dietary restrictions, and goals (fat loss, muscle gain, performance, wellness).
- **Real-Time Adjustments**: Syncing with wearables, recovery scores, and glucose monitors to shift calories or macros daily.
- **Food Preferences & Lifestyle**: Incorporating cultural diets, allergies, or time constraints.
- **Behavioral Cues**: Recognizing patterns (e.g., late-night snacking) and offering preemptive strategies.
- **Nutrient Balance**: Ensuring not just macros, but micronutrients and fiber are considered.

Benefits Over Traditional Meal Plans

- **Adaptability**: Plans evolve as your weight, body comp, and recovery change.
- **Personal Relevance**: Meals reflect your culture, taste preferences, and daily schedule.
- **Nutrient Precision**: AI balances not just calories, but protein, fats, carbs, and micronutrients.
- **Decision Relief**: Removes "What should I eat?" stress by narrowing choices to options that fit your goals.
- **Sustainability**: Flexibility reduces burnout compared to rigid diets.

Real-World Example

What Happened
A 40-year-old executive tried multiple diet templates — paleo, low-carb, intermittent fasting. Each worked short-term but failed long-term due to lifestyle conflicts.

What Changed
She adopted an AI-driven nutrition engine linked to her smartwatch. The system adjusted macros based on her training load and travel schedule, suggested culturally familiar meals, and offered quick substitutions when she missed targets.

Results
Instead of yo-yo dieting, she developed sustainable habits. Her energy improved, her body fat dropped gradually, and she stuck with the system for over a year.

What We Learn
Personalization and adaptability matter more than following the "perfect" diet. AI delivered both.

Common Pitfalls

- **Over-Complex Plans**: Some systems create meals too elaborate for busy users.
- **Ignoring User Feedback**: AI must allow overrides — not everyone wants salmon three nights in a row.
- **Database Limitations**: Missing local foods or cuisines can make plans less relevant.
- **Over-Reliance**: Users risk losing basic nutrition literacy if they blindly follow suggestions.

Tactical Best Practices

- **Start With Simplicity**: Use AI for 2–3 meals daily, then expand if needed.
- **Prioritize Variety**: Ask your engine to rotate proteins, veggies, and carbs weekly.
- **Add Your Own Favorites**: Input "go-to" meals so AI can integrate them.
- **Check Nutrient Gaps**: Use the AI's analysis to spot deficiencies (e.g., low magnesium).
- **Pair With Lifestyle Data**: Let training, sleep, and glucose feedback influence adjustments.

Final Thought

AI nutrition engines transform meal planning from rigid prescription into flexible partnership. By combining your biological signals, lifestyle, and preferences, they create meal plans that are not only precise but also practical. The result isn't just better nutrition — it's long-term consistency.

Next Steps

With meal planning personalized, the next frontier is convenience. In the following section, we'll explore **Grocery List Optimization With AI**, showing how these platforms streamline shopping by turning nutrition plans into efficient, cost-effective grocery strategies.

Grocery List Optimization with AI

Even the smartest meal plan fails if your kitchen isn't stocked with the right ingredients. This is where most people stumble: they start the week with a healthy plan, but by midweek they're missing key foods and default to takeout. Grocery shopping may seem simple, but it's the logistical backbone of every nutrition strategy.

AI takes the guesswork and inefficiency out of grocery planning. By linking directly to your meal plan, dietary preferences, and even local store inventories, AI can generate optimized grocery lists that save time, reduce waste, and ensure you always have the right foods on hand.

How AI Optimizes Grocery Lists

1. **Meal Plan Integration**
   - Converts your weekly meals into exact ingredient quantities.
   - Adjusts automatically if you swap meals or change portion sizes.
2. **Inventory Awareness**
   - Some platforms let you track pantry items. AI won't add foods you already have, reducing duplicate buys.
3. **Local Store Syncing**
   - Connects to grocery delivery apps or store catalogs to ensure items are available where you shop.

4. **Smart Substitutions**
   - Suggests alternatives if a food is unavailable (e.g., quinoa → brown rice) while preserving nutrition balance.
5. **Cost Optimization**
   - Highlights lower-cost equivalents or bulk-buy opportunities to save money without sacrificing quality.

Benefits of AI-Powered Grocery Lists

- **Time Savings**: No more scribbling lists or forgetting key items.
- **Reduced Waste**: Portion-based planning prevents overbuying perishable foods.
- **Consistency**: Keeps your kitchen aligned with your nutrition goals.
- **Budget Efficiency**: Identifies cost-friendly swaps and highlights seasonal produce.
- **Stress Reduction**: Transforms shopping from a chore into a streamlined process.

Real-World Example

What Happened
A busy family of four struggled to stick with healthier eating because grocery runs were chaotic. Foods spoiled, meals got skipped, and takeout became the fallback.

What Changed
They adopted an AI nutrition app that generated a weekly grocery list based on their meal plan and synced with their preferred supermarket. The app also suggested family-friendly swaps for picky eaters.

Results

Food waste dropped by 25%, grocery costs stabilized, and family meals became consistent. The parents reported less stress and fewer midweek "emergency" takeout orders.

What We Learn

Sustainability isn't just about willpower. It's about systems. AI turned grocery shopping into a support system, not a stumbling block.

Common Pitfalls

- **Over-Reliance on Deliveries**: May lead to less awareness of food quality if you never visit the store.
- **Database Gaps**: Some niche or cultural foods may not be recognized.
- **Rigid Substitutions**: AI may recommend impractical swaps unless you fine-tune preferences.
- **Ignoring Budget Settings**: Without cost filters, lists can skew toward expensive ingredients.

Tactical Best Practices

- **Sync to Your Meal Plan Weekly**: Don't rely on one-time lists; update as plans shift.
- **Mark Pantry Staples**: Teach the app what you already stock (e.g., olive oil, spices).
- **Set Budget and Store Preferences**: Guide AI to match your financial and logistical realities.
- **Use Substitutions Wisely**: Approve or override swaps based on taste and family needs.
- **Review Before Checkout**: Always do a quick scan to catch items you don't need.

Final Thought

AI grocery list optimization bridges the gap between planning and execution. It ensures your nutrition goals don't collapse under logistical friction, saving time, money, and effort while making healthy eating far more sustainable.

Next Steps
Meal prep isn't just about logistics — it's also about psychology. In the next section, we'll explore **Predicting Cravings and Substitution Strategies**, where AI helps anticipate weak points and offers smarter swaps before temptation derails progress.

Predicting Cravings and Substitution Strategies

No nutrition plan fails in theory — it fails in practice. And one of the biggest disruptors of consistency is **cravings.** Whether it's the 3 p.m. sugar urge at the office or the late-night pull toward salty snacks, cravings derail even the most disciplined people.

AI nutrition platforms are increasingly tackling this challenge head-on. By analyzing biometric data, eating patterns, and behavioral cues, these systems don't just track your cravings — they *predict* them. More importantly, they provide substitution strategies in real time, helping you stay aligned with your goals without feeling deprived.

How AI Predicts Cravings

- **Blood Sugar Patterns**: AI synced with CGMs detects when glucose dips are likely to trigger hunger.
- **Sleep and Stress Data**: Poor sleep and elevated stress increase cravings for quick-energy foods — AI can spot this.
- **Behavioral Logs**: Historical patterns (e.g., always craving sweets mid-afternoon) are factored into predictions.

- **Hormonal Cycles**: For women, AI can adjust recommendations based on menstrual phases linked to stronger cravings.
- **Time-of-Day Trends**: AI highlights windows of vulnerability and prepares proactive strategies.

Smart Substitution Strategies

Instead of simply saying "don't eat that," AI provides **actionable swaps** that satisfy the craving while preserving nutritional balance:

- **Sweet Cravings** → Swap candy for Greek yogurt with fruit or dark chocolate squares.
- **Salty Cravings** → Swap chips for roasted chickpeas or air-popped popcorn with olive oil.
- **Crunch Factor** → Swap cookies for apple slices with nut butter.
- **Energy Crashes** → Swap sugary drinks for sparkling water with electrolytes.
- **Comfort Eating** → Swap takeout pizza for a high-protein wrap with cheese and veggies.

AI learns what substitutions *you* actually enjoy, personalizing future recommendations.

Real-World Example

What Happened
A 35-year-old consultant repeatedly sabotaged her nutrition by indulging in sugary snacks during long workdays. She thought it was a lack of willpower.

What Changed
Her AI platform flagged low sleep and predicted an afternoon energy crash. At 2 p.m., it sent her a nudge: "Craving window ahead — try protein + fiber." She grabbed a pre-packed protein bar and sparkling water.

Results

Her cravings became manageable, her afternoon productivity improved, and she felt empowered instead of guilty.

What We Learn

Cravings aren't moral failures. They're predictable biological events. With foresight and substitutions, they can be managed intelligently.

Common Pitfalls

- **Rigid "Healthy Swaps"**: Substitutions that don't actually satisfy cravings can feel like punishment.
- **Ignoring Emotional Drivers**: Not all cravings are physiological — some are stress or boredom responses.
- **Overcomplicating Solutions**: Substitutions need to be quick, simple, and accessible.
- **All-or-Nothing Thinking**: Occasional indulgence isn't failure; AI can even help plan "flex" meals.

Tactical Best Practices

- **Stock Smart Alternatives**: Keep AI-recommended swaps available so you don't default to poor choices.
- **Track Craving Patterns**: Use the app to identify triggers and weak points in your routine.
- **Pair Protein + Fiber**: These combinations curb hunger better than sugar or fat alone.
- **Use AI Nudges**: Allow reminders during known craving windows.
- **Plan Indulgences**: Build small "flex foods" into your plan so cravings don't become binges.

Final Thought

Cravings are inevitable, but they don't have to derail progress. AI makes them predictable, manageable, and less emotional by offering real-time strategies. Instead of relying on brute willpower, you build a system where smart swaps keep you satisfied and on track.

Next Steps
With cravings under control, we now focus on **Balancing Macros with AI Recommendations** — where AI fine-tunes protein, carbs, and fats day by day to match your unique physiology and training demands.

Balancing Macros with AI Recommendations

Once you know how many calories you need, the next challenge is distributing them across **macronutrients** — protein, carbohydrates, and fats. Striking the right balance has a dramatic impact on body composition, performance, recovery, and even mood. Yet, finding that balance is notoriously tricky without support.

This is where AI steps in. By combining biometric data, training loads, and historical eating patterns, AI platforms can fine-tune your macro targets and adjust them dynamically. Instead of sticking to rigid ratios, you get a plan that adapts to *you* in real time.

Why Macro Balance Matters

- **Protein**: Supports muscle repair, satiety, and metabolism.
- **Carbohydrates**: Provide quick and sustainable energy, replenish glycogen, and regulate hormones.
- **Fats**: Support hormone health, brain function, and vitamin absorption.

The balance shifts based on your **goals**:

- Fat loss often means higher protein to preserve muscle.
- Muscle gain requires a calorie surplus with enough carbs to fuel training.
- Endurance sports need higher carb ratios for sustained energy.

How AI Balances Macros

1. **Adaptive Ratios**
   - AI recalculates macros based on training intensity, recovery markers, and even hormonal cycles.
2. **Meal Timing Adjustments**
   - Suggests higher carbs around workouts or more fats on low-activity days.
3. **Integration with Glucose & Wearables**
   - Real-time glucose data refines carb recommendations.
   - Wearable insights on sleep and recovery guide fat/protein shifts.
4. **Behavioral Feedback Loops**
   - If you consistently under-consume protein, AI flags it and suggests practical fixes (e.g., high-protein snacks).

Real-World Example

What Happened
A 29-year-old strength athlete plateaued despite training hard. His macros were fixed at 40% carbs, 30% protein, 30% fat, but his recovery lagged after heavy sessions.

What Changed
His AI nutrition app identified that post-leg-day glucose dips were leaving him under-fueled. It increased his carb target by 20% on training days and reduced fats slightly to balance calories.

Results

He recovered faster, added strength, and broke through his plateau within 6 weeks.

What We Learn

Fixed macro ratios don't respect day-to-day variability. AI-driven flexibility ensures nutrition matches training demands.

Common Pitfalls

- **Over-Fixation on Percentages**: 40/30/30 is a starting point, not a law.
- **Ignoring Recovery**: High training loads require adaptive carb intake.
- **Undereating Protein**: Still the most common mistake, especially for women.
- **Micromanaging Daily**: Obsessing over perfection discourages sustainability.

Tactical Best Practices

- **Anchor with Protein First**: Hit protein goals daily; let carbs and fats flex.
- **Cycle Carbs with Training**: Higher carbs on intense days, lower on rest days.
- **Use AI Nudges**: Let platforms remind you to adjust meals if you're off track.
- **Review Weekly Trends**: Focus on averages, not single-day fluctuations.
- **Stay Flexible**: Macro targets are guidelines, not shackles.

Final Thought

Balancing macros is both art and science. AI brings precision to the science — adjusting protein, carbs, and fats with context from your workouts, recovery, and daily habits. The result isn't just a "better diet" but a smarter, adaptive fuel system for your goals.

Next Steps
Not every diet follows a standard macro distribution. In the next section, we'll explore **AI Support for Special Diets (Keto, Vegan, Allergies)** — and how personalization engines help people thrive within unique dietary frameworks.

AI Support for Special Diets (Keto, Vegan, Allergies)

Nutrition is never one-size-fits-all. Beyond general macro balancing, many people follow **special diets** — whether by choice, cultural practice, medical need, or ethical belief. Historically, this made meal planning even harder because traditional apps and diet templates often ignored the unique restrictions and requirements of these eating styles.

AI nutrition engines are closing this gap. By incorporating dietary rules, preferences, and medical constraints into their algorithms, they generate meal plans and recommendations that honor restrictions *without sacrificing balance or variety.*

How AI Supports Special Diets

1. **Rule-Based Customization**
   o   AI engines filter out restricted foods (meat, dairy, gluten, nuts, etc.) and build plans only from compliant ingredients.
2. **Nutrient Gap Detection**
   o   Identifies common deficiencies in specific diets (e.g., B12 for vegans, electrolytes for keto) and suggests solutions.
3. **Smart Substitutions**
   o   Replaces restricted items with nutritionally similar alternatives (e.g., lentils instead of chicken for protein).

4. **Integration with Health Data**
   - o Syncs with wearables or CGMs to adjust special diets dynamically (e.g., refining carb intake for keto users).

Examples of AI in Action

- **Keto Diets**
  AI monitors carb intake closely, ensuring meals stay within 20–50g daily. It also adjusts fat/protein balance and suggests electrolyte-rich foods to prevent the "keto flu."
- **Vegan Diets**
  AI flags potential gaps (B12, iron, omega-3s, protein) and recommends fortified foods or plant-based combinations (e.g., rice + beans for complete proteins).
- **Food Allergies/Intolerances**
  Users input allergens (e.g., peanuts, shellfish, lactose). AI avoids risky foods while offering substitutes that preserve nutritional density.

Real-World Example

What Happened
A 25-year-old vegan athlete struggled to hit protein targets while training for triathlons. Traditional apps only recommended generic plant meals, often too low in key nutrients.

What Changed
Her AI nutrition app learned her preferences and built protein-rich vegan plans with lentils, edamame, tofu, and fortified products. It flagged her omega-3 deficiency and suggested flax, chia, and algae-based supplements.

Results
She boosted recovery, improved endurance, and avoided fatigue without abandoning her ethical food choices.

What We Learn
AI respects dietary frameworks while intelligently filling gaps —
something rigid plans rarely achieve.

Common Pitfalls

- **Over-Restriction**: Without AI, many people unintentionally narrow diets too much, leading to deficiencies.
- **Poor Substitutions**: Swaps that fit the diet but miss key nutrients (e.g., vegan junk food).
- **Ignoring Individual Response**: Keto works differently for everyone; AI helps track glucose and ketone responses.
- **Database Gaps**: Some apps lack global or culturally specific foods.

Tactical Best Practices

- **Input All Restrictions Clearly**: Allergies, intolerances, and ethical choices should be non-negotiable rules in the AI system.
- **Check for Nutrient Gaps**: Use AI reports to identify and address common deficiencies early.
- **Approve Substitutions**: Review AI-recommended swaps to ensure they align with your taste and lifestyle.
- **Pair With Biometrics**: Especially for restrictive diets, use wearables or lab work to validate health markers.
- **Keep Variety**: AI can rotate ingredients weekly to prevent monotony and ensure balance.

Final Thought

Special diets don't have to mean special struggles. AI simplifies the process by respecting restrictions, filling nutritional gaps, and providing real-time adaptability. Whether for medical necessity, ethical choice, or lifestyle preference, AI ensures your diet works *for you* — not against you.

Next Steps

In the following section, we'll dive into **Real-Time Adjustments Based on Feedback Loops** — where AI doesn't just set your plan once but continuously learns from your body's signals, adjusting nutrition and training in sync with your evolving needs.

Real-Time Adjustments Based on Feedback Loops

Traditional diets fail because they're static. They assume your body, routine, and energy needs are the same every day. In reality, your physiology is dynamic — influenced by stress, sleep, training, hormones, and countless environmental factors.

AI changes the game by creating **feedback loops**: systems where your data feeds into algorithms, which then adjust your nutrition plan in real time. Instead of being locked into a fixed schedule, your plan evolves with your life.

How Feedback Loops Work

1. **Data Collection**
   o Wearables, CGMs, smart scales, and food logs capture continuous input: sleep quality, recovery scores, glucose responses, weight changes, and more.
2. **Pattern Recognition**
   o AI identifies correlations: poor sleep → higher cravings, intense workouts → increased carb needs, stress → glucose spikes.
3. **Dynamic Adjustment**
   o Nutrition targets shift daily or weekly. Example: carbs rise after high-intensity training days, fats increase on rest days, protein stays steady.
4. **User Feedback**
   o The system learns from your choices. If you swap meals or skip snacks, AI recalibrates future recommendations without guilt or rigidity.

Why Real-Time Adjustment Matters

- **Personalization at Scale**: No two days look alike — your plan shouldn't either.
- **Faster Adaptation**: Stalls and plateaus are corrected before they become discouraging.
- **Sustainability**: Flexible adjustments prevent feelings of failure when life gets messy.
- **Peak Performance**: Aligns energy intake with recovery needs for consistent training output.

Real-World Example

What Happened
A 32-year-old corporate professional followed a strict macro plan but constantly missed targets on high-stress days with poor sleep. The mismatch led to fatigue and weekend overeating.

What Changed
Her AI-powered platform integrated wearable data. When her sleep was short, the system adjusted her carbs upward to prevent energy crashes and recommended magnesium-rich foods for recovery. On high-activity days, it boosted protein and carb intake.

Results
Her consistency improved, overeating episodes declined, and she felt energized instead of drained by her plan.

What We Learn
Flexibility beats rigidity. Real-time feedback loops allow nutrition to serve your body, not fight it.

Common Pitfalls

- **Ignoring Long-Term Trends**: Real-time changes are useful, but big-picture reviews are equally vital.

- **Data Quality Issues**: Inaccurate logging or faulty wearable readings can skew recommendations.
- **Overreacting Daily**: Small fluctuations shouldn't trigger extreme changes — balance is key.
- **Neglecting User Input**: AI can't account for preference shifts unless you provide feedback.

Tactical Best Practices

- **Prioritize Consistency in Data**: Weigh or log meals at similar times for clearer trends.
- **Review Weekly Reports**: Let AI show you patterns beyond daily adjustments.
- **Trust Flexibility**: Missing one target isn't failure — AI adapts around it.
- **Combine Objective + Subjective Feedback**: Input mood, energy, and hunger to refine AI recommendations.
- **Stay Educated**: Understand *why* adjustments happen, not just *what* they are.

Final Thought

AI-driven feedback loops bring nutrition into real life. Instead of rigid diets that demand you fit into them, adaptive systems mold around your body, lifestyle, and needs. This creates resilience, sustainability, and the freedom to keep moving forward without perfection.

Next Steps
With nutrition fully adaptive, it's time to see how AI revolutionizes movement. In **Chapter 6 – AI in Fitness Training Programs**, we'll explore how AI designs smarter workouts, balances training load, and personalizes exercise programming in ways no static plan ever could.

CHAPTER 6

AI in Fitness Training Programs

Adaptive Workout Design Based on Progress

In traditional training programs, workouts are often written weeks or even months in advance. While this gives structure, it also locks you into a plan that may not reflect your actual progress, recovery, or lifestyle shifts. The result? Programs that either stall or push you into injury.

AI-driven adaptive workout design changes this entirely. By continuously analyzing your performance, recovery, and physiological data, AI creates **living programs** that evolve with you. Every set, rep, and session can be fine-tuned to match your readiness and goals in real time.

How Adaptive Design Works

1. **Baseline Establishment**
   - The system starts with your fitness level, training history, and goals.
2. **Data Collection**
   - Wearables and workout logs track reps, weights, time, HR, HRV, VO_2 max, and perceived exertion.
3. **Trend Analysis**
   - AI detects when you're improving (lifting more weight, recovering faster) or regressing (plateaus, rising fatigue).
4. **Dynamic Adjustment**
   - Workouts are modified session by session:
     - If recovery is poor $\rightarrow$ lower intensity or switch to mobility work.
     - If strength is improving quickly $\rightarrow$ increase load or reps.
     - If endurance stalls $\rightarrow$ adjust intervals or recovery times.

Benefits of Adaptive Programming

- **Faster Progression**: Increases load or volume only when your body is ready.
- **Reduced Injury Risk**: Adjusts intensity when recovery signals are low.
- **Personalization**: Plans are unique to your progress, not a generic template.
- **Consistency**: Keeps training engaging and prevents boredom from static routines.
- **Efficiency**: Eliminates wasted time on workouts that don't match your current capacity.

Real-World Example

What Happened
A 42-year-old beginner started with a traditional 12-week strength plan. By week 5, the workouts felt too easy, but the plan didn't change. Motivation dropped, and progress stalled.

What Changed
She switched to an AI workout app that adapted her program weekly. When she progressed faster than expected, the app increased weights and added complexity. When she slept poorly, it reduced intensity and prescribed mobility drills.

Results
She stayed consistent, avoided injury, and built strength faster than with her static plan.

What We Learn
Adaptation keeps training aligned with reality, not just theory.

Common Pitfalls

- **Over-Adjustment**: Daily changes can overwhelm users who prefer structure.
- **Ignoring Long-Term Goals**: Adaptation should fit within a bigger progression framework.
- **Data Quality Issues**: Inaccurate inputs (e.g., mislogged weights or missed wearable syncs) skew results.
- **User Resistance**: Some athletes resist AI adjustments, sticking to "their way" instead.

Tactical Best Practices

- **Set Clear Long-Term Goals**: Strength, endurance, fat loss — adaptation should serve these outcomes.
- **Trust the Process, but Review Weekly**: Don't obsess over daily changes; trends matter more.
- **Provide Feedback**: Rate difficulty honestly so AI can calibrate effectively.
- **Mix Flexibility and Structure**: Allow AI to adapt the details while keeping broader routines consistent (e.g., "3 strength days + 2 cardio days").
- **Use Data + Intuition**: If the AI says "go hard" but your body feels off, listen to yourself first.

Final Thought

AI-powered adaptive workout design makes training dynamic, personal, and sustainable. By adjusting to your actual performance and readiness, it ensures you keep progressing without burning out or stalling. It's like having a coach who's watching every rep — and rewriting your plan in real time.

Next Steps
With adaptive design covered, we now move to a cutting-edge
frontier: **Computer Vision for Form Correction (AI Video
Analysis)** — where your phone or wearable camera doubles as a
virtual trainer, ensuring your movements are safe and effective.

Computer Vision for Form Correction (AI Video Analysis)

One of the greatest challenges in training without a coach is **form.**
Poor technique doesn't just slow progress — it dramatically
increases the risk of injury. For decades, proper form correction
required an in-person trainer's eye. Today, **AI-powered computer
vision** is bringing that same feedback into your living room or gym.

By using your smartphone camera, connected sensors, or wearable
motion trackers, computer vision analyzes your movements in real
time. The AI compares your biomechanics against optimal patterns,
then gives instant cues to help you correct errors.

How Computer Vision Works

1. **Movement Capture**
   o A phone camera or wearable sensor records your
     motion during an exercise.
2. **Pose Estimation**
   o AI maps key body points (joints, limbs, angles) into a
     skeletal model.
3. **Pattern Comparison**
   o Your movement is compared against a library of
     optimal form patterns.
4. **Real-Time Feedback**
   o On-screen cues (e.g., "straighten back," "deepen
     squat," "adjust elbow angle") are delivered instantly.

Benefits of AI Form Correction

- **Immediate Feedback**: Corrects mistakes in the moment, not days later.
- **Injury Prevention**: Identifies unsafe angles or loads before they cause harm.
- **Confidence for Beginners**: Provides reassurance without needing to hire a trainer immediately.
- **Data for Long-Term Improvement**: Logs form errors over time, showing patterns and progress.
- **Scalability**: Offers coaching access to millions of people at low cost.

Real-World Example

What Happened
A 30-year-old remote worker started lifting at home with YouTube videos as her guide. Over time, she developed recurring lower back pain.

What Changed
She tried an AI-powered form correction app. The system flagged her excessive spinal flexion during deadlifts and cued her to brace her core and hinge at the hips.

Results
Her pain subsided, her lifts improved, and she felt confident training independently.

What We Learn
Form feedback doesn't need to be intimidating or inaccessible. AI provides an affordable safety net.

Common Pitfalls

- **Camera Positioning**: Poor angles reduce accuracy; AI needs clear sightlines.
- **Over-Reliance**: Users may ignore how their body *feels* in favor of chasing "perfect" AI scores.
- **Context Blindness**: AI may not recognize individual anatomy variations or mobility limitations.
- **Connectivity Needs**: Real-time analysis can lag without strong internet or device power.

Tactical Best Practices

- **Set Up Proper Angles**: Place your phone at hip height and ~3–4 meters away for most lifts.
- **Use Feedback Selectively**: Focus on 1–2 key corrections per session, not perfection.
- **Pair With Awareness**: Check in with how your body feels alongside AI cues.
- **Start With Foundational Movements**: Squats, deadlifts, push-ups — these benefit most from AI feedback.
- **Review Progress Over Time**: Use AI reports to see if errors are decreasing.

Final Thought

Computer vision makes quality coaching accessible at scale. While it won't replace a human trainer's nuance, it dramatically raises the safety and effectiveness of solo training. With real-time corrections and logged progress, AI ensures you're not just moving more — you're moving better.

Next Steps
Now that we've seen how AI protects form, we'll explore **AI-Generated Training Splits and Cycles** — how algorithms design weekly and monthly training structures that balance recovery, progression, and long-term performance goals.

AI-Generated Training Splits and Cycles

Designing a workout split — how you divide training across the week — and structuring training cycles over months has traditionally been the work of coaches. Done well, it balances progress and recovery. Done poorly, it leads to burnout, plateaus, or injury.

AI now automates this process with precision. By analyzing your goals, recovery signals, and training history, AI creates **adaptive splits and periodized cycles** that evolve with your performance. Instead of guessing between "bro splits" or "push/pull/legs," you get a program designed for *your* physiology.

How AI Designs Training Splits

1. **Input Goals**
   o Fat loss, hypertrophy, strength, endurance, or sport-specific performance.
2. **Assess Resources**
   o Available equipment, weekly time commitment, and training environment.
3. **Analyze Readiness Data**
   o Sleep quality, HRV, and muscle recovery scores inform intensity placement.
4. **Generate Splits**
   o Examples:
      ▪ **3 Days/Week** → Full-body or push/pull/legs.
      ▪ **4–5 Days/Week** → Upper/lower or strength + hypertrophy mixes.
      ▪ **Athletic Focus** → Skill, conditioning, and recovery distribution.
5. **Adjust Weekly**
   o If recovery drops, AI shifts to deloads or lighter sessions.
   o If performance improves, AI adds progression or variety.

How AI Builds Training Cycles

Training isn't just about weeks — it's about *cycles*. AI uses **periodization** strategies that scale over time:

- **Microcycles (1 week)**: Day-to-day structure.
- **Mesocycles (4–6 weeks)**: Focused training blocks (e.g., hypertrophy, endurance).
- **Macrocycles (3–6 months)**: Long-term progression toward a major goal (e.g., marathon, body recomposition).

AI adapts cycles dynamically:

- If fatigue markers rise → adjust volume or intensity.
- If progress accelerates → shorten cycle and advance sooner.
- If injury risk appears → extend recovery block.

Real-World Example

What Happened
A 36-year-old lawyer tried to follow a classic bodybuilding split but frequently missed sessions due to work. This led to imbalances and stalled progress.

What Changed
His AI training app condensed his split into a 3-day full-body program, adjusting intensity based on his recovery scores. Over 12 weeks, it automatically periodized into hypertrophy, strength, and deload phases.

Results
He gained muscle, avoided injury, and stuck to his plan despite an unpredictable schedule.

What We Learn
AI doesn't force your life to fit the plan. It builds a plan around your life.

Common Pitfalls

- **Rigid Thinking**: Users expect fixed splits instead of letting AI adapt.
- **Chasing Volume**: More isn't always better; AI balances load intelligently.
- **Ignoring Recovery Data**: Splits only work if recovery inputs are tracked and respected.
- **One-Size Templates**: Not all apps have deep AI — some just recycle generic splits.

Tactical Best Practices

- **Be Honest With Time Commitment**: Overestimating leads to missed workouts and broken plans.
- **Sync Recovery Metrics**: HRV, sleep, and soreness should guide adjustments.
- **Trust Adaptation**: Let AI shorten or lengthen cycles based on your progress.
- **Mix Goals Over Time**: Strength, endurance, and mobility should rotate for balance.
- **Review Monthly**: Use AI summaries to see cycle progression and goal alignment.

Final Thought

AI-generated splits and cycles bring structure without rigidity. They honor long-term progression while adjusting in real time to recovery and lifestyle. This blend of planning and adaptability creates the consistency most people struggle to achieve.

Next Steps
Having covered splits and cycles, the next section explores **Recovery Tracking and Adjustment of Intensity** — where AI doesn't just prescribe workouts but ensures you're training at the right effort for your body's current state.

Recovery Tracking and Adjustment of Intensity

One of the most overlooked elements in fitness isn't how hard you train — it's how well you recover. Progress happens not during the workout itself but in the hours and days afterward, when your body repairs tissue, restores energy, and adapts. Ignoring recovery is one of the fastest ways to plateau, burn out, or get injured.

AI solves this by making recovery measurable. Through wearables, biometrics, and user input, AI can track how ready your body is for training and automatically adjust workout intensity. This turns training into a **dynamic cycle** of stress and adaptation — not a blind push toward exhaustion.

Key Recovery Metrics AI Monitors

- **Heart Rate Variability (HRV)**: A strong indicator of nervous system readiness. Low HRV often signals stress or fatigue.
- **Resting Heart Rate (RHR)**: Elevated RHR can suggest poor recovery, illness, or overtraining.
- **Sleep Quality and Quantity**: Deep sleep and REM stages strongly influence recovery capacity.
- **Muscle Soreness and Fatigue**: Logged manually or inferred from movement quality.
- **Daily Stress Levels**: Detected through wearable sensors or self-reports.

How AI Adjusts Intensity

1. **Session Scaling**
   - On low-recovery days, intensity may drop from heavy lifting to mobility work or lighter cardio.
   - On high-recovery days, AI may increase volume or load for optimal progress.

2. **Adaptive Training Zones**
   o Heart rate or power targets shift dynamically based on readiness.
3. **Cycle Adjustments**
   o If poor recovery persists, AI may recommend a deload week or recovery block.
4. **Lifestyle Feedback**
   o AI can suggest earlier bedtimes, hydration targets, or stress-reducing habits if poor recovery trends are detected.

Real-World Example

What Happened
A 39-year-old amateur triathlete trained six days per week, constantly fatigued, and eventually hit a performance plateau.

What Changed
His AI-enabled wearable tracked HRV and flagged chronic under-recovery. The system reduced intensity on flagged days, recommended sleep adjustments, and inserted structured recovery sessions.

Results
His energy rebounded, training quality improved, and he set a new personal best in his next race — despite doing *slightly fewer workouts.*

What We Learn
More training isn't always better. Smarter training — guided by recovery — produces better results.

Common Pitfalls

- **Ignoring Recovery Scores**: Many users treat AI recovery warnings as "optional."
- **Chasing Consistency Over Health**: Pushing through fatigue for streaks often backfires.

- **One-Dimensional Metrics**: Relying only on sleep or HRV without context can mislead.
- **Assuming Rest = Weakness**: Recovery is performance fuel, not laziness.

Tactical Best Practices

- **Review Recovery Daily**: Use readiness scores as a guide, not a dictator.
- **Plan Intensity Waves**: Let AI scale sessions instead of aiming for maximum effort every time.
- **Pair Data With Feel**: Combine objective recovery scores with your subjective energy levels.
- **Respect Deload Weeks**: Scheduled breaks are not setbacks — they're accelerators.
- **Address Root Causes**: If recovery scores are chronically low, look at sleep, stress, and nutrition, not just training.

Final Thought

AI doesn't just design workouts — it acts as a guardrail, ensuring training pushes you forward without pushing you over the edge. By tracking recovery and adjusting intensity, it removes guesswork and creates a sustainable cycle of stress and adaptation.

Next Steps
Once the foundation of recovery is in place, the next opportunity is making training fun and engaging. In the following section, we'll explore **Gamification Through AI Challenges** — how AI uses competition, rewards, and progress tracking to turn consistency into a game you actually want to play.

Gamification Through AI Challenges

One of the hardest parts of fitness isn't knowing what to do — it's staying motivated long enough to do it consistently. This is why so many gyms see a January rush followed by a February drop-off. AI-powered platforms tackle this issue by introducing **gamification**: using game-like elements such as challenges, badges, leaderboards, and streaks to keep people engaged.

When powered by AI, gamification goes beyond superficial rewards. It adapts challenges to your fitness level, predicts when your motivation is waning, and delivers the right nudge at the right time.

How AI Gamifies Training

- **Personalized Challenges**
  AI sets challenges that are achievable yet motivating — for example, increasing daily steps by 10% or hitting a recovery score streak.
- **Adaptive Progression**
  Instead of static "30-day challenges," AI scales goals as you improve, ensuring they stay within reach but still push growth.
- **Social Competition**
  Leaderboards and team challenges allow for friendly rivalry, adjusted for fairness so beginners and advanced users both stay engaged.
- **Reward Systems**
  Points, badges, or streaks reinforce consistency — and AI rewards behaviors that match *your* goals, not arbitrary metrics.
- **Behavioral Nudges**
  If AI notices a drop in activity or motivation, it may deliver a small, winnable challenge to rebuild momentum.

Benefits of AI Challenges

- **Motivation Boost**: Makes progress feel rewarding in real time.
- **Consistency Builder**: Streaks and small wins reinforce daily action.
- **Community Connection**: Group challenges add accountability and fun.
- **Psychological Engagement**: Turns workouts from "chores" into achievements.
- **Personalized Growth**: Challenges scale with you, preventing boredom or burnout.

Real-World Example

What Happened
A 28-year-old struggled to stick with her fitness routine beyond three weeks. She lacked accountability and found workouts repetitive.

What Changed
She joined an AI-powered fitness app with adaptive challenges. The system started with a 7-day streak challenge, rewarded her for hitting hydration goals, and later introduced team-based competitions synced to her wearable.

Results
She built a 90-day streak, improved fitness measurably, and felt motivated by earning "badges" for both training and recovery milestones.

What We Learn
AI gamification works because it makes consistency fun and progress visible — not because it invents new exercises, but because it changes the *experience*.

Common Pitfalls

- **Overemphasis on Points**: Chasing badges can lead to ignoring true progress markers.
- **Unrealistic Challenges**: Poorly set goals (too hard or too easy) reduce engagement.
- **Comparison Traps**: Social leaderboards may discourage if not well-calibrated.
- **Short-Term Thinking**: Gamification should build habits, not just deliver temporary motivation.

Tactical Best Practices

- **Start Small**: Choose 1–2 simple challenges to build consistency before layering more.
- **Personalize Metrics**: Let AI align rewards with your actual goals (e.g., recovery, strength, or endurance).
- **Mix Solo and Social**: Alternate personal streaks with group competitions for variety.
- **Celebrate Recovery Wins**: Don't just reward workouts — reward smart rest as well.
- **Track Real Progress Too**: Use AI dashboards to measure strength, endurance, or body comp alongside gamified badges.

Final Thought

AI challenges make fitness sticky. By transforming effort into a game, they keep people engaged long after motivation would normally fade. Done right, gamification isn't about distraction — it's about building momentum, accountability, and joy into the fitness journey.

Next Steps

With gamification boosting motivation, the next question is about guidance: **Virtual Trainers vs. In-Person Coaches.** In the following section, we'll explore where AI trainers shine, where humans are still essential, and how the two can complement each other.

Virtual Trainers vs. In-Person Coaches

The rise of AI-driven fitness apps and virtual trainers has sparked a critical question: *can technology replace the role of a human coach?* The answer isn't simple, because both virtual trainers and in-person coaches bring unique strengths to the table. Understanding the difference helps individuals choose the model — or hybrid — that works best for them.

What Virtual Trainers Offer

- **Accessibility**: Available 24/7, whether you're at home, traveling, or in the gym.
- **Personalized Programs at Scale**: AI adapts workouts to your recovery, progress, and schedule.
- **Cost-Effectiveness**: Fraction of the price of private coaching.
- **Data-Driven Decisions**: Uses wearables, recovery scores, and biometrics to refine plans.
- **Consistency**: Always ready, never distracted, and impossible to "miss an appointment."

What In-Person Coaches Provide

- **Real-Time Form Correction**: Subtle adjustments AI can miss, especially with complex lifts.
- **Emotional Support**: Motivation, empathy, and accountability tailored to your personality.
- **Contextual Coaching**: A coach can adapt a session if you're stressed, injured, or short on time.

- **Human Connection**: For many, the relationship itself is the biggest driver of consistency.
- **Creativity**: Coaches can improvise workouts based on available equipment or mood.

The Hybrid Future

Rather than replacing one another, the smartest approach is combining both:

- **Virtual Trainers as the Base**: AI delivers daily programming, tracks recovery, and handles adjustments.
- **In-Person Coaches as Specialists**: Step in to refine technique, provide motivation, and adapt to life's nuances.
- **Shared Data**: Coaches can access AI-collected data, making their interventions more precise.

Real-World Example

What Happened
A 33-year-old professional used an AI training app but struggled with squat form, leading to knee pain.

What Changed
She booked monthly in-person sessions with a trainer who corrected her movement. Between sessions, she relied on her AI app for adaptive workouts.

Results
Her pain resolved, her performance improved, and her program felt more sustainable than with either approach alone.

What We Learn
The best solution wasn't choosing AI *or* a coach — it was leveraging both.

Common Pitfalls

- **Over-Reliance on Tech**: AI can't catch every nuance of human movement or mindset.
- **Assuming Coaches Are Obsolete**: Good coaches offer value beyond program writing.
- **High Costs of Exclusivity**: Relying only on in-person coaching may be financially unsustainable.
- **Fragmentation**: Without integration, AI and human coaching can feel disconnected.

Tactical Best Practices

- **Use AI for Consistency**: Let it handle daily decisions and progress tracking.
- **Seek Human Input Periodically**: Even occasional coaching sessions pay dividends.
- **Share Your Data**: Provide trainers with AI insights (HRV, sleep, performance) for context.
- **Blend Accountability Systems**: Use AI for reminders and streaks, while relying on a coach for motivation and emotional support.
- **Reassess Regularly**: Your needs may shift — flexibility is the key.

Final Thought

Virtual trainers and in-person coaches aren't competitors — they're partners. AI excels at data, adaptability, and affordability, while humans excel at empathy, context, and connection. The most effective path forward isn't choosing one over the other but blending both to create a system that is precise, supportive, and sustainable.

Next Steps

With coaching models explored, we now move to **Chapter 7 – Monitoring Progress with AI**, where we'll examine how data-driven feedback, visualizations, and trend analysis help you measure results more effectively than ever before.

CHAPTER 7

Monitoring Progress with AI

Tracking Weight and Body Fat Trends

Progress in fitness and nutrition is rarely linear. The scale might dip one week, spike the next, and plateau for days in between. For many people, these fluctuations lead to frustration, self-doubt, and even abandonment of their goals. But with the help of AI, weight and body fat trends can be analyzed with context, turning noisy numbers into clear, actionable insights.

Why Weight Alone Isn't Enough

- **Daily Fluctuations**: Hydration, sodium, hormones, and digestion can swing weight by several pounds.
- **Muscle vs. Fat**: A scale can't distinguish between fat loss and lean muscle gain.
- **Misleading Plateaus**: You may be improving body composition even when weight stalls.

This is why tracking **both weight and body fat percentage** provides a more accurate picture of progress.

How AI Analyzes Weight & Body Fat

1. **Data Smoothing**
   o AI averages daily weigh-ins to eliminate short-term noise, showing true long-term trends.
2. **Pattern Recognition**
   o Detects cycles (e.g., menstrual fluctuations) and removes them from misleading results.
3. **Integration with Activity & Nutrition**
   o Links weight and fat changes to training load, recovery, and calorie/macronutrient intake.
4. **Predictive Insights**
   o Forecasts plateaus or rebounds before they happen, recommending adjustments early.

5. **Contextual Reporting**
   o Highlights fat loss vs. muscle gain to prevent discouragement when the scale moves slowly.

Real-World Example

What Happened
A 37-year-old tracked weight daily and became discouraged when it stalled for 10 days despite perfect adherence.

What Changed
His AI app smoothed the data and revealed a clear downward fat-loss trend hidden by water retention from high-sodium meals. It reassured him the plan was working.

Results
He stuck with his program, eventually dropping 15 pounds of fat while preserving lean muscle.

What We Learn
Raw numbers can mislead. AI turns short-term noise into long-term clarity.

Common Pitfalls

- **Obsessing Over Daily Weigh-Ins**: Leads to emotional rollercoasters.
- **Ignoring Body Fat Data**: Only looking at weight misses the bigger picture.
- **Using Inconsistent Tools**: Switching scales or methods creates unreliable readings.
- **Expecting Linear Progress**: Progress almost never follows a straight line.

Tactical Best Practices

- **Weigh in daily, but focus weekly**: Use AI to smooth daily noise into weekly trends.
- **Track body fat alongside weight**: Smart scales or photo-based AI tools provide more insight than weight alone.
- **Stay consistent**: Weigh at the same time each day (morning, fasted) for accuracy.
- **Pair data with performance**: Use strength, endurance, and recovery metrics to complete the picture.
- **Review monthly trends**: Long-term changes matter more than daily shifts.

Final Thought

Weight and body fat tracking can be frustrating without context. AI smooths the noise, identifies patterns, and delivers clarity that prevents discouragement. Instead of reacting to every fluctuation, you learn to trust the bigger picture — and keep moving forward with confidence.

Next Steps
With weight and fat trends in perspective, we'll now explore **AI for Visual Body Transformation Analysis** — how computer vision and progress photos combine with AI to track changes your eyes might miss.

AI for Visual Body Transformation Analysis

When it comes to fitness progress, numbers tell part of the story — but visuals often tell it better. Many people rely on progress photos, but comparing images over time is subjective and prone to bias. Lighting, angles, and even posture can distort the truth.

AI-powered visual body transformation analysis takes this process further. By applying computer vision, it removes human bias and translates photos into objective, measurable insights. This makes it possible to see *true* progress that the mirror (or scale) might not reveal.

How AI Visual Analysis Works

1. **Image Capture**
   o Users upload photos or 3D scans taken under consistent conditions.
2. **Pose Detection & Mapping**
   o AI identifies body landmarks (shoulders, waist, hips, thighs, etc.) and builds a skeletal map.
3. **Comparison Over Time**
   o Measurements like waist-to-hip ratio, posture alignment, and muscle symmetry are tracked against past images.
4. **Highlighting Changes**
   o AI overlays before-and-after images, emphasizing subtle fat loss, muscle growth, or posture improvements.
5. **Integration with Metrics**
   o Visual progress is synced with weight, body fat, and workout performance to create a complete picture.

Why This Matters

- **Objectivity**: Removes bias that comes from judging photos emotionally.
- **Motivation**: Visualizing progress keeps people engaged during plateaus.
- **Precision**: Identifies subtle shifts — like posture or muscle tone — that scales miss.
- **Holistic Tracking**: Combines aesthetics with health markers for balanced insights.

Real-World Example

What Happened
A 29-year-old was frustrated by minimal scale movement after 8 weeks of training. She felt discouraged and thought she wasn't making progress.

What Changed
Her AI progress app compared day-1 and week-8 photos. It highlighted reduced waist circumference, improved posture, and visible muscle definition.

Results
She realized she was losing fat and gaining muscle simultaneously. Seeing measurable change in her body shape renewed her motivation.

What We Learn
The mirror can lie. AI helps reveal the quiet, steady progress happening beneath the surface.

Common Pitfalls

- **Inconsistent Photo Conditions**: Different lighting, clothing, or poses reduce accuracy.
- **Over-Focus on Aesthetics**: Visuals matter, but they're only part of overall health.
- **Privacy Concerns**: Sensitive photos require secure storage and encryption.
- **Unrealistic Comparisons**: Comparing against social media "ideals" instead of your own baseline.

Tactical Best Practices

- **Standardize Photos**: Same lighting, same angles, same time of day.
- **Track Monthly, Not Daily**: Visible changes require time; avoid impatience.
- **Combine With Metrics**: Use alongside weight, fat %, and performance for full context.
- **Secure Your Data**: Only use platforms with strong privacy protections.
- **Focus on Trends**: Look at long-term shape changes, not short-term fluctuations.

Final Thought

AI visual analysis bridges the gap between how you feel, how you look, and how you perform. By removing guesswork, it transforms progress photos from a subjective exercise into a reliable tool for motivation and accountability.

Next Steps
Beyond aesthetics, fitness is about function. In the next section, we'll cover **Performance Metrics: Strength, Endurance, Flexibility** — and how AI tracks these pillars of fitness to create a well-rounded picture of progress.

Performance Metrics: Strength, Endurance, Flexibility

While weight loss or physique changes often get the spotlight, **true fitness is multidimensional.** Strength, endurance, and flexibility are equally important markers of progress — and often the ones that make the biggest difference in how you feel and perform daily.

AI is transforming the way these metrics are tracked, shifting from vague self-assessments ("I feel stronger") to precise, adaptive measurements that evolve with you.

Tracking Strength with AI

- **Wearable Integration**: Sensors in smartwatches or gym equipment measure bar speed, rep quality, and total training load.
- **Form & Reps Detection**: Computer vision apps count reps, evaluate tempo, and assess range of motion.
- **Adaptive Benchmarking**: AI adjusts strength targets based on recent progress (e.g., suggesting a 5 lb increase after consistent performance).
- **Trend Analysis**: Instead of focusing on one lift, AI tracks total strength volume across major movements.

Tracking Endurance with AI

- **Heart Rate Zones**: AI analyzes your ability to sustain intensity across zones (aerobic vs. anaerobic).
- **VO$_2$ Max Estimates**: Wearables measure cardiovascular efficiency and update it automatically as fitness improves.
- **Recovery Curves**: AI monitors how quickly heart rate returns to baseline after exertion — a key endurance marker.
- **Adaptive Workouts**: Endurance sessions shift intensity based on real-time readiness.

Tracking Flexibility with AI

- **Range-of-Motion Analysis**: Camera-based AI apps measure joint angles during stretches or lifts.
- **Symmetry Checks**: AI highlights imbalances (e.g., tighter left hip vs. right).
- **Progressive Programming**: Suggests mobility drills tailored to problem areas.
- **Integration With Recovery**: Flexibility scores are factored into recovery and injury risk analysis.

Real-World Example

What Happened
A 41-year-old focused only on weight loss. Although she lost pounds, she still felt weak, inflexible, and easily fatigued.

What Changed
Her AI fitness app began tracking strength lifts, endurance intervals, and flexibility assessments. She saw clear improvements in barbell squats, VO_2 max, and hamstring mobility — even when the scale stalled.

Results
Her motivation shifted from chasing weight to celebrating performance gains. She became stronger, fitter, and more resilient overall.

What We Learn
Progress isn't just visible in the mirror. Performance markers reveal improvements that redefine what "fit" really means.

Common Pitfalls

- **Over-Focusing on One Metric**: Chasing strength while neglecting endurance or flexibility creates imbalances.
- **Inconsistent Testing**: Skipping regular assessments skews progress tracking.
- **Misusing Wearables**: Data is useless if not contextualized.
- **Neglecting Function**: Aesthetic goals can overshadow meaningful functional gains.

Tactical Best Practices

- **Test Regularly**: Schedule strength, endurance, and flexibility benchmarks every 4–6 weeks.
- **Balance Your Training**: Use AI programming that integrates all three domains.

- **Celebrate Non-Scale Wins**: PRs, mile times, and mobility milestones matter as much as body comp.
- **Use Trend Data**: AI helps you see gradual progress instead of obsessing over single results.
- **Integrate With Recovery**: Align training intensity with readiness to avoid overtraining.

Final Thought

Strength, endurance, and flexibility are the real markers of resilience. AI makes them measurable, trackable, and motivational by showing progress in areas that often go unnoticed. Together, these metrics define a healthier, more functional body — not just a lighter one.

Next Steps
To tie it all together, the next section will focus on **Automated Progress Reports** — how AI consolidates data across weight, visuals, and performance into easy-to-read updates that keep you informed and accountable.

Automated Progress Reports

One of the most frustrating parts of a fitness journey is figuring out whether all your effort is actually working. Spreadsheets, manual logs, and scattered notes rarely give the full picture. That's why many people feel lost — they can't see the forest for the trees.

AI solves this problem with **automated progress reports**. By consolidating data from wearables, workouts, nutrition logs, and body composition tools, AI creates clear, visual reports that show exactly where you're improving, where you're stalling, and what adjustments might be needed.

What Automated Reports Include

- **Body Metrics**: Weight trends, body fat %, muscle mass.
- **Performance Gains**: Strength PRs, VO₂ max, endurance improvements.
- **Nutrition Tracking**: Average calorie intake, macro consistency, micronutrient gaps.
- **Recovery Insights**: HRV, sleep quality, readiness scores.
- **Behavioral Patterns**: Craving windows, missed workouts, adherence streaks.

Why They Matter

- **Clarity**: Summarizes hundreds of data points into a single, digestible snapshot.
- **Accountability**: Weekly or monthly reports reinforce consistency.
- **Motivation**: Highlighting progress in multiple areas keeps users engaged beyond just scale changes.
- **Decision Support**: AI doesn't just report data — it recommends next steps (e.g., "increase daily protein by 15g").

Real-World Example

What Happened
A 34-year-old accountant tracked workouts and food separately but felt confused about whether he was progressing.

What Changed
His AI platform began delivering weekly reports. They showed his weight was stable, but strength had risen by 8% and his recovery scores had improved. The report also flagged inconsistent protein intake as a weak spot.

Results

He shifted focus from weight alone to overall performance and nutrition consistency. Motivation returned, and he continued making steady progress.

What We Learn

Progress isn't always obvious day to day. Automated reports make it undeniable.

Common Pitfalls

- **Information Overload**: Reports packed with too many metrics can overwhelm.
- **Focusing Only on Positives**: Sugarcoated reporting doesn't drive improvement.
- **Ignoring Recommendations**: Reports are useless if no action follows.
- **Short-Term Thinking**: Weekly reports are helpful, but long-term comparisons (quarterly, yearly) matter too.

Tactical Best Practices

- **Choose Frequency Wisely**: Weekly for accountability, monthly for big-picture analysis.
- **Highlight 3–4 Key Metrics**: Don't drown in data — focus on what matters most to your goals.
- **Follow AI Recommendations**: Treat reports as a playbook, not just a scoreboard.
- **Compare Across Timeframes**: Look at monthly and quarterly progress, not just weekly shifts.
- **Celebrate Wins**: Use reports to acknowledge both major and subtle improvements.

Final Thought

Automated progress reports transform scattered numbers into meaningful narratives. By making progress visible and actionable, AI eliminates doubt, boosts confidence, and creates a clear roadmap for continued success.

Next Steps
With progress reports in place, the next focus is **Early Detection of Plateaus** — how AI identifies stalled progress before it becomes discouraging, and what strategies it recommends to break through.

Early Detection of Plateaus

Every fitness journey eventually hits a **plateau** — the frustrating point where progress slows or stops altogether. For many, this is where motivation crumbles, old habits return, and goals are abandoned. Plateaus aren't just about effort; they're about adaptation. The body becomes more efficient at a given workload, requiring new stimuli to keep progressing.

AI offers a solution by detecting plateaus earlier than humans typically can. By analyzing data trends across weight, performance, and recovery, AI flags subtle signs of stagnation before they become major roadblocks — giving you the chance to adjust strategy proactively.

How AI Detects Plateaus

1. **Trend Analysis**
   o AI smooths short-term fluctuations and identifies when progress curves flatten.
2. **Cross-Metric Correlation**
   o If weight stalls but strength improves, that's not a plateau — it's recomposition.
   o If *all* metrics flatline (weight, strength, endurance), the system recognizes stagnation.

3. **Timeframe Monitoring**
   o AI knows the difference between a natural short-term stall (a few days) and a true plateau (several weeks).
4. **Behavioral Tracking**
   o Missed workouts, declining sleep, or inconsistent nutrition patterns can explain why progress paused.

Benefits of Early Detection

- **Saves Motivation**: Prevents frustration by explaining why results slowed.
- **Guides Adjustments**: AI suggests new training loads, nutrition tweaks, or recovery changes.
- **Protects from Overtraining**: Sometimes plateaus signal fatigue, not laziness.
- **Supports Long-Term Growth**: Keeps progress moving by avoiding prolonged stalls.

Real-World Example

What Happened
A 44-year-old man lost 15 pounds quickly, then saw no scale change for three weeks. He felt defeated and considered quitting.

What Changed
His AI progress app flagged the stall as a plateau. It highlighted increased strength gains and suggested a 5% calorie reduction paired with an added cardio session.

Results
Weight loss resumed, and he realized the plateau wasn't failure — it was feedback.

What We Learn
AI reframes plateaus not as dead-ends, but as checkpoints that require recalibration.

Common Pitfalls

- **Mistaking Fluctuations for Plateaus**: A week of no change isn't a plateau. AI helps avoid overreaction.
- **Blaming Willpower Alone**: Plateaus are biological, not just behavioral.
- **One-Dimensional Tracking**: Looking only at the scale can mask progress in strength or endurance.
- **Delaying Adjustments**: Waiting months to course-correct wastes valuable time.

Tactical Best Practices

- **Track Multiple Metrics**: Weight, strength, endurance, and body fat together paint a fuller picture.
- **Trust AI Alerts**: If flagged, review recommendations instead of guessing.
- **Adjust in Small Steps**: Minor tweaks (5–10% changes) are usually enough to break a plateau.
- **Stay Patient**: True plateaus last weeks, not days — consistency matters most.
- **Reframe as Progress**: Plateaus signal that your body adapted, which means growth has already occurred.

Final Thought

Plateaus aren't failures; they're signals. With AI, you no longer need to wonder if you've stalled — you'll know, and you'll have a clear roadmap for breaking through. By detecting stagnation early, AI keeps you engaged, motivated, and progressing toward your goals.

Next Steps
Breaking a plateau is just one step. In the next section, we'll explore **Using Feedback to Reset Goals** — how AI leverages progress data to refine your targets and keep your fitness journey aligned with your evolving capabilities.

Using Feedback to Reset Goals

Fitness is not a straight line. As you progress, the goals you started with may no longer reflect your current reality. Maybe you set out to lose 20 pounds, but halfway through, you realize you've gained muscle and your ideal target has shifted. Or perhaps you aimed for a 10K run, but along the way discovered a passion for strength training.

AI helps you navigate this evolution by turning raw progress data into **feedback loops** that refine and reset your goals. Instead of clinging to outdated targets, you're guided toward objectives that are realistic, motivating, and aligned with your body's actual performance.

How AI Uses Feedback to Refine Goals

1. **Progress Analysis**
   o Tracks trends in weight, strength, endurance, recovery, and adherence.
   o Highlights whether you're ahead, on track, or behind relative to your initial goal.
2. **Contextual Adjustments**
   o If fat loss slows but strength surges, AI may suggest shifting focus to body recomposition instead of scale weight.
3. **Goal Reset Recommendations**
   o AI proposes new milestones based on your rate of progress (e.g., aiming for 12% body fat instead of chasing an arbitrary number).
4. **Motivation Calibration**
   o Aligns goals with what excites you — whether that's performance, aesthetics, or health markers.

Why Resetting Goals Matters

- **Keeps Motivation High**: Achievable, relevant goals maintain momentum.
- **Prevents Burnout**: Unrealistic expectations are a recipe for failure.
- **Supports Adaptation**: Fitness evolves; so should your targets.
- **Promotes Sustainability**: Long-term success comes from flexible, living goals.

Real-World Example

What Happened
A 31-year-old set a goal to drop 30 pounds. After losing 18, the scale slowed, but her AI app showed major muscle and strength gains.

What Changed
The system recommended resetting her target to 5 more pounds of fat loss paired with a performance milestone: a personal best in deadlift.

Results
She stopped obsessing over the last 12 pounds, celebrated visible muscle, and gained confidence in strength training.

What We Learn
Goals aren't fixed endpoints — they're checkpoints. AI helps you pivot instead of quit.

Common Pitfalls

- **Clinging to Arbitrary Numbers**: Sticking with outdated targets can demoralize.
- **Ignoring Progress Beyond the Scale**: Weight alone misses strength, mobility, and endurance gains.

- **Resetting Too Often**: Constant goal-switching undermines focus; balance flexibility with consistency.
- **Not Celebrating Milestones**: Failing to acknowledge wins before moving the goalposts.

Tactical Best Practices

- **Review Goals Quarterly**: Let AI summarize your progress and suggest refinements.
- **Shift from Outcome to Process Goals**: From "lose 20 lbs" to "hit protein target 80% of days."
- **Include Performance Metrics**: Add strength, endurance, or mobility alongside physique goals.
- **Stay Realistic but Challenging**: Goals should stretch you, not overwhelm you.
- **Celebrate Achievements**: Mark each reset as progress, not failure.

Final Thought

Fitness isn't static, and your goals shouldn't be either. AI provides the clarity and adaptability to reset targets based on feedback, keeping you motivated and aligned with your evolving body and lifestyle. The journey becomes less about chasing arbitrary numbers and more about sustainable growth.

Next Steps
With adaptive goal setting in place, we move into **Chapter 8 – Overcoming Plateaus with AI**, where we'll explore in depth how AI strategies break through the toughest sticking points and keep your progress moving forward.

CHAPTER 8

Overcoming Plateaus with AI

Identifying Causes of Stalled Progress

Every fitness journey eventually runs into a wall. Workouts that once delivered results stop working. The scale refuses to budge. Strength or endurance plateaus. These stalls, while frustrating, are part of the natural adaptation process — your body becomes more efficient at handling the stress you've been applying.

The key isn't to panic, but to understand *why* progress has stalled. This is where AI excels. By scanning across multiple data streams, AI can pinpoint the likely cause of a plateau — whether it's nutritional, training-related, or recovery-driven — and guide you toward the right fix.

Common Causes of Stalled Progress

1. **Nutritional Misalignment**
   - Calorie intake no longer matches goals (e.g., metabolic adaptation reduces calorie burn).
   - Macro imbalances limit energy or muscle growth.
   - Hidden calories or inconsistent tracking skew results.
2. **Training Inefficiency**
   - Workouts lack progressive overload.
   - Too much repetition of the same program without variation.
   - Excessive cardio or overemphasis on one type of training.
3. **Recovery Deficits**
   - Inadequate sleep, poor stress management, or insufficient rest days.
   - Chronic fatigue suppressing performance.
4. **Psychological & Behavioral Factors**
   - Motivation dips, adherence falls, or emotional eating creeps back in.
   - Skipping "small" habits like hydration or stretching undermines results.

How AI Detects These Causes

- **Cross-Metric Correlation**: AI links stalled weight loss to inconsistent nutrition logs or stagnant performance metrics.
- **Pattern Recognition**: Identifies trends like reduced sleep preceding strength plateaus.
- **Behavior Tracking**: Notices drops in adherence (missed workouts, skipped meals).
- **Predictive Modeling**: Forecasts when adaptation will likely cause a stall based on past cycles.

Real-World Example

What Happened
A 40-year-old male saw great results in the first 12 weeks of training but then hit a wall. Despite consistent workouts, weight loss stopped.

What Changed
His AI app analyzed his wearable and nutrition data. It found that his calorie intake had crept up slightly, recovery scores were dropping due to short sleep, and his workouts had not changed in over 8 weeks.

Results
The AI flagged the plateau and suggested a small calorie adjustment, improved sleep hygiene, and a new workout split. Progress resumed within two weeks.

What We Learn
Plateaus rarely have one cause. AI uncovers the *combination* of factors behind stalled progress.

Common Pitfalls

- **Blaming the Wrong Variable**: Many assume training is the issue when nutrition or sleep is the real culprit.
- **Changing Too Much Too Soon**: Overhauling diet and training simultaneously makes it hard to see what worked.
- **Ignoring Lifestyle Factors**: Stress, hydration, and even work schedules can derail progress.
- **Expecting Linear Results**: Bodies adapt in cycles, not straight lines.

Tactical Best Practices

- **Use AI Analysis Weekly**: Let systems flag potential stalls before they become long-term.
- **Start With the Smallest Fix**: Tweak one factor (calories, training volume, or recovery) instead of overhauling everything.
- **Cross-Check Metrics**: If progress stalls, look at nutrition + training + recovery together.
- **Stay Objective**: Rely on data, not emotions, when progress slows.
- **Review Cycles Regularly**: Adjust programs every 4–6 weeks to prevent stagnation.

Final Thought

Plateaus are not failures — they're feedback. By identifying the causes of stalled progress, AI transforms frustration into clarity. Instead of guessing or quitting, you gain a roadmap to break through and keep advancing toward your goals.

Next Steps
Once causes are identified, the next move is action. In the following section, we'll explore **AI Suggestions for Dietary Tweaks**, showing how small, intelligent adjustments can reignite fat loss, muscle gain, or performance improvements.

AI Suggestions for Dietary Tweaks

When progress slows, nutrition is often the first place to look. Even small mismatches between intake and goals can stall fat loss, muscle gain, or energy levels. The challenge for most people is knowing exactly *what* to change — without overcorrecting or making their diet unsustainable.

AI simplifies this process. Instead of guessing, it analyzes your nutrition logs, biometric responses, and performance data, then recommends precise, minimal adjustments that get results moving again. These tweaks are often subtle — and that's the point. The best changes are the ones that fit seamlessly into your life.

Types of AI-Driven Dietary Adjustments

1. **Calorie Calibration**
   - Detects when your intake is too high (stalling fat loss) or too low (slowing metabolism and recovery).
   - Suggests modest adjustments (e.g., -150 calories/day) instead of extreme cuts.
2. **Macro Rebalancing**
   - Identifies protein shortfalls and nudges intake upward for muscle retention or growth.
   - Adjusts carbs around workouts to fuel training and recovery.
   - Increases healthy fats if hormonal or energy markers flag imbalances.
3. **Meal Timing Optimization**
   - Suggests shifting carb intake earlier or later based on glucose and energy data.
   - Recommends protein distribution across meals for better satiety and recovery.
4. **Nutrient Gap Filling**
   - Flags deficiencies in vitamins, minerals, or fiber.
   - Suggests specific foods or supplements to address gaps without overhauling the diet.

5. **Behavioral Adjustments**
   o Detects skipped meals or evening overeating patterns.
   o Provides substitution strategies or reminder nudges at vulnerable times.

Real-World Example

What Happened
A 35-year-old woman plateaued after losing 12 pounds. She felt fatigued, and her strength stopped improving.

What Changed
Her AI app scanned her logs and noted that her protein intake averaged only 0.6g per pound of body weight, well below optimal. It also identified that late-night snacks were pushing her calorie intake slightly above her target.

Results
The system recommended increasing daily protein by 30g and reducing evening snacks by ~200 calories. Within two weeks, fat loss resumed, and energy levels improved.

What We Learn
Plateaus don't require drastic diet overhauls. Small, AI-driven tweaks can make all the difference.

Common Pitfalls

- **Overcorrecting**: Slashing 500+ calories creates fatigue and rebounds.
- **Ignoring Protein**: Many users under-consume protein, slowing results.
- **Changing Too Many Variables**: Makes it impossible to know what worked.
- **Focusing Only on Calories**: Macronutrient balance and timing are equally important.

Tactical Best Practices

- **Trust Small Tweaks**: Start with 5–10% changes in calories or macros.
- **Review Weekly**: Let AI summarize whether changes are working.
- **Focus on Protein First**: Hitting protein goals solves most plateau issues.
- **Match Carbs to Activity**: Use higher-carb meals on training days, lower-carb on rest days.
- **Log Consistently**: AI can only optimize what it can measure.

Final Thought

Dietary tweaks don't have to be complicated or extreme. AI's strength lies in precision: identifying the smallest possible changes that unlock continued progress. By combining data with personalization, it ensures your nutrition works *with* you — not against you.

Next Steps
Nutrition is just one part of the equation. In the following section, we'll explore **Adaptive Workout Reshuffling** — how AI reconfigures training loads, splits, and exercise selection to keep your body challenged and progressing.

Adaptive Workout Reshuffling

Just as diets can stall progress, so can workouts. Following the same exercises, sets, and routines for too long eventually leads to **adaptation** — your body becomes efficient, and the growth stimulus disappears. Traditionally, lifters and athletes relied on intuition or cookie-cutter programs to "mix things up." But this often meant either too much change (losing progress) or too little (remaining stuck).

AI introduces a smarter solution: **adaptive workout reshuffling.** Instead of random variety, AI selectively rotates exercises, rep ranges, or intensity based on your performance trends, recovery markers, and progression history. The goal isn't novelty for its own sake — it's targeted disruption that reignites growth without derailing momentum.

How AI Reshuffles Training

1. **Exercise Rotation**
   - Swaps in variations of staple lifts (e.g., barbell bench → dumbbell bench → push-ups with weighted vest).
   - Prevents overuse injuries while keeping muscle groups challenged.
2. **Volume & Intensity Shifts**
   - Modifies sets, reps, or weights to balance stimulus and recovery.
   - Example: Dropping rep count but adding load when strength stalls.
3. **Split Adjustments**
   - Shuffles training frequency (upper/lower, push/pull, full-body) based on fatigue and availability.
4. **Tempo & Rest Tweaks**
   - Recommends slower eccentric reps or shorter rest periods to increase stimulus without adding more weight.
5. **Readiness-Driven Substitutions**
   - If recovery scores are low, AI swaps heavy lifts for mobility or conditioning.
   - If energy is high, AI slots in a higher-intensity session.

Benefits of Adaptive Reshuffling

- **Breaks Through Plateaus**: Introduces enough novelty to shock adaptation.
- **Protects From Injury**: Rotates stress points before overuse develops.

- **Keeps Workouts Engaging**: Prevents boredom by offering variety without chaos.
- **Balances Load and Recovery**: Adjusts intensity instead of blindly pushing harder.
- **Maximizes Long-Term Growth**: Ensures consistent progression without burnout.

Real-World Example

What Happened
A 29-year-old male lifter stalled on bench press for three months. Despite pushing harder, his numbers refused to climb.

What Changed
His AI app detected stagnation and reshuffled his workouts by swapping in incline dumbbell presses, dips, and pause reps. It also reduced overall pressing volume for one week before reintroducing heavier loads.

Results
Within four weeks, he broke through his plateau, hitting a new bench press personal best.

What We Learn
Plateaus often need intelligent variety — not more of the same.

Common Pitfalls

- **Random Changes**: Constantly switching exercises without strategy creates chaos, not progress.
- **Ignoring Recovery Data**: Reshuffling volume without considering fatigue worsens stalls.
- **Overcomplicating Workouts**: Too much novelty makes tracking and progression harder.
- **Forgetting Fundamentals**: Core lifts should stay central — variety supports, not replaces them.

Tactical Best Practices

- **Rotate Every 4–6 Weeks**: Allow enough time for adaptation before reshuffling.
- **Keep Core Movements Consistent**: Use squats, deadlifts, presses, and pulls as anchors.
- **Add, Don't Overhaul**: Introduce 1–2 new elements at a time.
- **Use Recovery to Guide**: Let AI recovery scores dictate intensity swaps.
- **Review Progress After Changes**: Reassess performance within 2–3 weeks to measure impact.

Final Thought

Adaptive workout reshuffling is the antidote to stagnation without the chaos of random programming. By intelligently adjusting exercises, intensity, and structure, AI ensures your body stays challenged — breaking through plateaus while protecting long-term consistency.

Next Steps
Beyond training variety, another hidden plateau-buster lies in lifestyle. In the next section, we'll explore **Sleep and Stress Analysis for Breakthroughs** — how AI uncovers recovery bottlenecks and mental strain that silently sabotage progress.

Sleep and Stress Analysis for Breakthroughs

Sometimes, the cause of a plateau isn't diet or exercise at all — it's what happens in the hours between workouts. Poor sleep and unmanaged stress silently sabotage progress by impairing recovery, altering hormones, and draining motivation. Even if training and nutrition are "perfect," these hidden factors can block results.

AI platforms are uniquely equipped to reveal these blind spots. By analyzing sleep quality and stress markers, they show how lifestyle factors contribute to stalled progress — and more importantly, they recommend practical strategies to unlock breakthroughs.

How AI Tracks Sleep

- **Sleep Stages**: Wearables detect light, deep, and REM sleep patterns.
- **Consistency**: AI flags irregular bedtimes and wake-up times that disrupt circadian rhythm.
- **Sleep Efficiency**: Measures time in bed vs. actual rest.
- **Recovery Link**: Cross-references sleep with HRV, RHR, and workout performance.

How AI Tracks Stress

- **Physiological Markers**: HRV, resting heart rate, and breathing patterns signal stress load.
- **Behavioral Inputs**: Missed workouts, inconsistent nutrition, or logged mood data.
- **Lifestyle Patterns**: AI detects correlations between work hours, screen time, and stress levels.
- **Integration with Recovery**: Combines stress analysis with sleep data to assess readiness.

Why Sleep and Stress Matter for Plateaus

- **Hormonal Impact**: Poor sleep elevates cortisol, which hinders fat loss and recovery.
- **Energy Levels**: Fatigue reduces workout intensity and adherence.
- **Recovery Bottleneck**: Stress keeps the body in "fight-or-flight," impairing adaptation.
- **Craving Amplification**: Both factors increase appetite for high-calorie foods.

Real-World Example

What Happened
A 38-year-old runner plateaued despite consistent mileage and careful nutrition.

What Changed
His AI wearable flagged poor sleep consistency (averaging <6 hours) and high daily stress scores. The system recommended a bedtime routine, screen-time reduction, and adding 10 minutes of breathwork daily.

Results
Within a month, his recovery scores improved, he felt more energetic, and his running pace dropped by nearly 20 seconds per mile.

What We Learn
Sometimes the "invisible" factors — sleep and stress — are the real plateau breakers.

Common Pitfalls

- **Blaming Training Alone**: Many assume workouts are the problem when lifestyle factors are to blame.
- **Ignoring Sleep Consistency**: Catching up on weekends isn't the same as nightly quality sleep.
- **Downplaying Stress**: Treating stress as "normal" instead of addressing it.
- **Band-Aid Fixes**: Supplements or stimulants without solving the root causes.

Tactical Best Practices

- **Track Sleep Consistently**: Use AI wearables to monitor stages and total rest.

- **Prioritize Bedtime Routines**: Consistent wind-down habits improve quality.
- **Integrate Stress Management**: Meditation, walks, or breathwork logged into your platform.
- **Review Weekly Reports**: Let AI highlight correlations between stress, sleep, and stalled progress.
- **Act on Red Flags**: If readiness scores dip, scale back training intensity until sleep and stress normalize.

Final Thought

Sleep and stress are often the missing puzzle pieces in breaking through plateaus. AI brings them out of the shadows, showing you not just how much they matter but exactly what to do about them. By optimizing recovery outside the gym, you create the conditions for breakthroughs inside it.

Next Steps
With sleep and stress addressed, AI can take things a step further: **Predictive Modeling for Habit Adjustments** — using your historical data to anticipate setbacks and recommend proactive lifestyle changes before plateaus even occur.

Predictive Modeling for Habit Adjustments

The most powerful use of AI in fitness isn't just analyzing where you are today — it's forecasting where you might get stuck tomorrow. **Predictive modeling** allows AI to anticipate habit breakdowns and plateaus before they happen, then recommend proactive adjustments to keep you on track.

Instead of reacting to stalls after weeks of frustration, predictive systems help you "course-correct" in real time. Think of it as a coach who doesn't just tell you what went wrong, but sees the problem coming and gives you tools to prevent it.

How Predictive Modeling Works

1. **Historical Data Analysis**
   - AI reviews your past training, nutrition, recovery, and lifestyle trends.
   - Identifies triggers for skipped workouts, overeating, or stalled results.
2. **Behavioral Correlation**
   - Connects events like poor sleep, late work nights, or travel with lapses in consistency.
3. **Pattern Forecasting**
   - Projects when habits are likely to break down (e.g., weekends, high-stress weeks, holidays).
4. **Proactive Suggestions**
   - Offers preemptive strategies: quick workouts for travel days, low-effort meals for busy weeks, or stress relief prompts during known pressure cycles.

Benefits of Predictive Modeling

- **Prevents Plateaus Before They Start**: Keeps small lapses from snowballing.
- **Personalized Prevention**: Targets your unique weak spots, not generic advice.
- **Builds Resilience**: Helps you create contingency plans for real-life disruptions.
- **Saves Motivation**: Fewer stalls mean less frustration and more consistency.

Real-World Example

What Happened
A 30-year-old professional frequently derailed her nutrition plan during business trips. Each time, she lost weeks of progress.

What Changed
Her AI platform detected the pattern after three trips and predicted upcoming challenges. It suggested pre-ordering healthy airport meals, packing protein snacks, and replacing long workouts with 20-minute hotel room sessions.

Results
She stayed consistent through travel, avoided major regressions, and hit her fat-loss target ahead of schedule.

What We Learn
By anticipating obstacles, predictive modeling turns "I'll get back on track later" into "I never left the track."

Common Pitfalls

- **Over-Engineering**: Too many predictive nudges can feel overwhelming.
- **Neglecting User Input**: AI predictions work best when paired with your feedback.
- **False Alarms**: Not every deviation is a crisis; balance predictions with flexibility.
- **Short-Term Focus**: Long-term habit trends matter more than occasional blips.

Tactical Best Practices

- **Review Forecasts Weekly**: Use AI habit predictions like a calendar check-in.
- **Plan for "Risk Windows"**: Anticipate disruptions (holidays, busy seasons) with simplified routines.
- **Accept Small Adjustments**: Don't aim for perfection; prioritize consistency.
- **Give Feedback**: Confirm when AI predictions are right or wrong to improve accuracy.
- **Celebrate Prevention**: Track avoided lapses as victories, not just workouts completed.

Final Thought

Predictive modeling turns fitness from reactive to proactive. By forecasting risks and suggesting small habit adjustments, AI empowers you to stay consistent even when life gets messy. Instead of fighting setbacks, you stay one step ahead — and that's how long-term success is built.

Next Steps
Of course, data isn't everything. Plateaus aren't just physical; they're psychological. In the next section, we'll explore **Psychological Support via AI Coaching Apps** — how digital coaching tools provide encouragement, accountability, and mindset shifts when motivation dips.

Psychological Support via AI Coaching Apps

Breaking through a plateau isn't always about food, workouts, or even recovery. Sometimes, the real challenge is **mental.** Frustration, self-doubt, or boredom can quietly erode consistency long before physical progress halts. This is why psychological support is becoming a core feature of modern AI coaching apps — helping people stay motivated, accountable, and resilient through the ups and downs of their fitness journey.

How AI Provides Psychological Support

1. **Motivational Nudges**
   o Timely reminders that celebrate small wins, highlight streaks, or encourage effort after setbacks.
2. **Behavioral Reinforcement**
   o Positive reinforcement (badges, progress highlights) keeps users focused on consistency, not perfection.
3. **Cognitive Reframing**
   o AI reframes "failure" as feedback, reminding you that plateaus are part of growth.

4. **Adaptive Communication**
   o Uses your logged mood, energy, or adherence data to deliver context-aware encouragement (e.g., "Low energy today? Let's aim for a lighter session instead of skipping.").
5. **Community Integration**
   o Many apps combine AI coaching with peer challenges or group accountability for a stronger psychological boost.

Why This Matters for Plateaus

- **Reduces Frustration**: Keeps motivation alive when results aren't immediately visible.
- **Promotes Resilience**: Encourages you to push through setbacks instead of quitting.
- **Normalizes Struggle**: Reminds users that stalls and dips are part of every journey.
- **Encourages Sustainable Habits**: Shifts focus from short-term results to long-term growth.

Real-World Example

What Happened
A 27-year-old hit a plateau in fat loss and considered abandoning her program. Her progress reports felt discouraging.

What Changed
Her AI coaching app began sending supportive nudges: highlighting her improved sleep, strength PRs, and streak consistency. It reframed her "plateau" as body recomposition and suggested a small adjustment in her nutrition.

Results
Instead of quitting, she stayed engaged, broke through the plateau, and built healthier long-term habits.

What We Learn

Sometimes the right words at the right time matter as much as the right workout or diet tweak.

Common Pitfalls

- **Over-Reliance on AI Encouragement**: Motivational nudges help, but shouldn't replace intrinsic drive.
- **Generic Messaging**: If support feels robotic, it loses impact.
- **Ignoring Emotional Nuance**: AI can miss deeper psychological struggles that require human coaching or therapy.
- **Short-Term Cheerleading**: Encouragement must be paired with actionable strategies.

Tactical Best Practices

- **Engage With the App Daily**: Use nudges and journaling features to keep accountability high.
- **Track Mood & Energy**: Give AI better context for personalized support.
- **Celebrate Non-Scale Wins**: Let AI highlight strength, recovery, and habit streaks.
- **Pair With Human Support**: Use AI for daily nudges but lean on friends, groups, or coaches for deeper accountability.
- **Stay Reflective**: Treat AI prompts as cues to pause, assess, and reset mindset.

Final Thought

Psychological resilience is the fuel that drives long-term consistency. By delivering motivation, reframing setbacks, and celebrating small wins, AI coaching apps act as a constant companion during the toughest moments. While they don't replace human empathy, they provide timely support that can make the difference between giving up and pushing through.

Next Steps

With plateaus now tackled both physically and mentally, we move into **Chapter 9 – Nutrition Optimization Beyond Dieting**, where we'll explore how AI shifts the conversation from short-term diets to long-term nutritional strategies that support energy, health, and performance for life.

CHAPTER 9

Nutrition Optimization Beyond Dieting

AI and Micronutrient Gap Detection

Most people think about calories and macros — protein, carbs, and fats — when they consider nutrition. But the real foundation of health lies in **micronutrients**: vitamins, minerals, and trace elements that support everything from energy production to immune defense. Deficiencies here don't just stall progress; they can quietly undermine mood, performance, and long-term health.

The challenge? Micronutrient gaps are hard to detect without lab tests, and most nutrition trackers either ignore them or treat them as afterthoughts. This is where AI brings a new level of precision. By analyzing your food logs, wearable data, and lifestyle inputs, AI can highlight **hidden deficiencies** and suggest strategies to correct them before they become serious issues.

How AI Detects Micronutrient Gaps

1. **Dietary Intake Analysis**
   o Scans logged foods against comprehensive nutrition databases.
   o Identifies which vitamins and minerals fall consistently below recommended levels.
2. **Pattern Correlation**
   o Links fatigue, poor recovery, or cravings with potential deficiencies (e.g., low magnesium correlating with poor sleep quality).
3. **Wearable & Biomarker Integration**
   o Syncs with devices that track sleep, stress, and recovery to spot symptoms tied to nutrient gaps.
   o Some platforms connect with lab results for direct biochemical feedback.
4. **Predictive Modeling**
   o Anticipates seasonal or lifestyle-based gaps (e.g., vitamin D deficiency risk in winter).

Why This Matters

- **Performance Optimization**: Adequate micronutrients improve recovery, strength, and endurance.
- **Disease Prevention**: Deficiencies raise risks for chronic conditions over time.
- **Energy & Mood**: Many mood and energy dips link back to vitamin or mineral gaps.
- **Personalization**: Needs vary widely by gender, age, activity, and lifestyle — AI accounts for these nuances.

Real-World Example

What Happened
A 34-year-old athlete logged consistent nutrition but struggled with restless sleep and frequent muscle cramps.

What Changed
Her AI platform flagged low magnesium and potassium intake. It recommended adding leafy greens, nuts, and electrolyte supplementation post-training.

Results
Within weeks, her sleep improved, cramps subsided, and workout recovery accelerated.

What We Learn
Small micronutrient gaps can have outsized impacts — and AI makes them visible.

Common Pitfalls

- **Overreliance on Apps Alone**: Not all AI platforms have robust micronutrient databases.
- **Assuming Perfect Accuracy**: Logging errors or incomplete food data can skew results.

- **Ignoring Bioavailability**: Not all nutrients are absorbed equally from different foods.
- **Skipping Medical Input**: AI insights should complement, not replace, blood tests or professional advice.

Tactical Best Practices

- **Log Food Consistently**: Even imperfect logging gives AI more accurate detection power.
- **Use Wearable Feedback**: Pair nutrient tracking with recovery and sleep data for context.
- **Prioritize Whole Foods**: Aim to fill gaps through food first before supplementation.
- **Review Seasonal Risks**: Vitamin D, hydration minerals, and iron are common recurring gaps.
- **Confirm with Testing**: Use lab work to validate AI predictions when possible.

Final Thought

Micronutrients may be "small," but their role is enormous. AI's ability to scan diet patterns, cross-reference symptoms, and predict deficiencies brings clarity to an area most people ignore. By making invisible gaps visible, AI empowers you to optimize health, energy, and performance from the inside out.

Next Steps
Detection is only half the equation. In the following section, we'll explore **AI Supplementation Recommendations** — how intelligent systems suggest precise, safe, and personalized supplements to fill those gaps without waste or guesswork.

AI Supplementation Recommendations

Once micronutrient gaps are identified, the next challenge is deciding how to close them. Should you eat more whole foods? Add a supplement? Which one, at what dose, and when? Most people guess — or worse, follow generic supplement stacks marketed to the masses. This often leads to wasted money, redundant products, or even overdosing certain vitamins and minerals.

AI helps cut through this noise by delivering **personalized supplementation strategies.** Instead of blindly recommending a "one-size-fits-all" multivitamin, AI integrates your nutrition logs, biometrics, lifestyle, and even lab results to recommend what *you* actually need — nothing more, nothing less.

How AI Recommends Supplements

1. **Gap Identification**
   o Uses food logs and biomarker data to confirm which nutrients are consistently low.
2. **Food-First Prioritization**
   o Suggests dietary solutions before recommending supplements (e.g., add salmon before omega-3 capsules).
3. **Personalized Dosage**
   o Recommends specific doses based on weight, gender, age, and activity level — not generic RDAs.
4. **Timing Optimization**
   o Suggests when to take supplements for best absorption (e.g., magnesium at night for sleep, iron away from caffeine).
5. **Safety Checks**
   o Flags potential overdoses from overlapping supplements (e.g., vitamin D from both a multivitamin and standalone capsule).

Why This Matters

- **Precision**: Avoids unnecessary supplementation and focuses only on real needs.
- **Cost Efficiency**: Eliminates spending on products that don't support your goals.
- **Safety**: Reduces risks of overdosing or harmful interactions.
- **Performance Optimization**: Ensures your body has exactly what it needs to recover, adapt, and perform.

Real-World Example

What Happened
A 42-year-old man took a generic multivitamin daily but still felt fatigued.

What Changed
His AI platform analyzed his logs and recovery data, then suggested discontinuing the multivitamin (which overdosed him on certain nutrients) and instead focusing on targeted vitamin D and magnesium supplementation.

Results
His fatigue eased, recovery improved, and his supplement routine became simpler and cheaper.

What We Learn
Less is more. AI helps eliminate the guesswork and clutter from supplementation.

Common Pitfalls

- **Over-Supplementation**: "More is better" thinking can backfire with fat-soluble vitamins or minerals.
- **Ignoring Food Sources**: Supplements should complement, not replace, whole foods.

- **Assuming AI Alone Is Enough**: Blood work and professional input are still essential for long-term accuracy.
- **Fad Products**: AI should prioritize essentials, not trendy powders with little evidence.

Tactical Best Practices

- **Confirm With Testing**: Use blood panels to verify AI recommendations when possible.
- **Start With Essentials**: Protein, vitamin D, omega-3, magnesium, and electrolytes are common foundational needs.
- **Personalize Timing**: Pair fat-soluble vitamins with meals; take sleep-supporting minerals at night.
- **Avoid Redundancy**: Check overlap if you're using multiple products.
- **Review Quarterly**: Needs change with seasons, training cycles, and goals.

Final Thought

Supplements should fill gaps, not replace real food or act as a magic solution. AI ensures they're used intelligently: personalized, precise, and always grounded in your unique data. This turns supplementation from a guessing game into a science-backed tool for optimal health and performance.

Next Steps
With micronutrients and supplements optimized, hydration becomes the next frontier. In the following section, we'll explore **Personalizing Hydration Strategies**, where AI fine-tunes water and electrolyte intake to your body, environment, and activity levels.

Personalizing Hydration Strategies

Hydration is often oversimplified into "drink eight glasses of water a day." While well-meaning, this advice ignores the fact that hydration needs vary dramatically from person to person — and even from day to day. Factors like training load, climate, body size, sweat rate, and diet all shape how much water and electrolytes you truly need.

AI brings precision to hydration by analyzing your individual data and creating **personalized strategies** that adapt in real time. This ensures you're not just drinking enough water, but also maintaining the right electrolyte balance for performance, recovery, and health.

How AI Personalizes Hydration

1. **Baseline Assessment**
   - Considers body weight, activity level, climate, and dietary intake.
   - Identifies hydration risks (e.g., high caffeine use or low fruit/vegetable intake).
2. **Wearable Integration**
   - Tracks sweat rate, body temperature, and fluid loss during workouts.
   - Syncs with exercise intensity and environmental conditions (heat, humidity).
3. **Electrolyte Balance**
   - Detects patterns of fatigue, cramps, or poor recovery linked to sodium, potassium, or magnesium deficits.
   - Suggests targeted electrolyte replacement, not just water.
4. **Real-Time Adjustments**
   - Recommends hydration strategies before, during, and after workouts.
   - Pushes reminders when dehydration risks spike (e.g., hot weather runs).

Why Personalized Hydration Matters

- **Performance**: Even mild dehydration can reduce endurance, strength, and mental sharpness.
- **Recovery**: Proper hydration accelerates nutrient delivery and muscle repair.
- **Health**: Prevents kidney strain, headaches, and long-term health complications.
- **Individual Differences**: A marathon runner in Florida needs more fluids and electrolytes than a desk worker in London.

Real-World Example

What Happened
A 29-year-old cyclist experienced recurring cramps during long summer rides despite drinking plenty of water.

What Changed
His AI platform tracked sweat rate and sodium loss via a connected wearable. It recommended electrolyte drinks with precise sodium/potassium ratios instead of plain water.

Results
Cramps disappeared, performance improved, and recovery time shortened.

What We Learn
Hydration isn't just about water — electrolyte balance is equally critical.

Common Pitfalls

- **Overhydration**: Drinking too much water without electrolytes can dilute sodium levels, leading to hyponatremia.
- **Generic Guidelines**: Following "8 cups per day" ignores personal variability.

- **Neglecting Electrolytes**: Water alone isn't enough for athletes or hot climates.
- **Reactive Instead of Proactive**: Waiting until you feel thirsty often means you're already dehydrated.

Tactical Best Practices

- **Weigh Before and After Workouts**: AI can use the difference to estimate sweat loss.
- **Use Hydration Reminders**: Let AI nudge you at intervals matched to your activity and environment.
- **Balance Fluids and Electrolytes**: Pair water with sodium, potassium, and magnesium, especially for endurance or heat exposure.
- **Adjust Seasonally**: Increase fluids in summer and when training volume spikes.
- **Log Subjective Feedback**: Note fatigue, headaches, or cramps — AI can link them to hydration.

Final Thought

Personalized hydration is about more than avoiding thirst — it's about optimizing energy, recovery, and resilience. With AI guiding intake based on real-world data, you move beyond generic advice and ensure your body is truly supported under every condition.

Next Steps
With hydration dialed in, the next layer of optimization lies inside the gut. In the following section, we'll explore **AI Insights on Gut Health and Digestion** — how AI helps decode the complex role of the microbiome in energy, recovery, and long-term wellness.

AI Insights on Gut Health and Digestion

The gut is often called the "second brain," and for good reason. It influences everything from nutrient absorption and immune health to mood and energy regulation. Yet, digestive health is one of the most misunderstood and overlooked aspects of nutrition. Many people struggle with bloating, irregular digestion, or food intolerances without clear answers — problems that can quietly stall progress and reduce quality of life.

AI is now helping to make gut health more measurable and actionable. By combining dietary data, wearable inputs, and in some cases microbiome testing, AI platforms can identify patterns that point to digestive imbalances and provide personalized strategies to improve gut function.

How AI Supports Gut Health

1. **Food Symptom Tracking**
   - Links dietary intake with logged symptoms like bloating, discomfort, or fatigue.
   - Identifies trigger foods (e.g., dairy, gluten, highly processed items).
2. **Microbiome Data Integration**
   - Some AI platforms analyze gut microbiome sequencing tests.
   - Suggests foods that promote beneficial bacteria and overall gut balance.
3. **Digestive Efficiency Insights**
   - Cross-references nutrient intake with energy levels, recovery quality, and inflammation markers.
   - Detects when absorption may be impaired.
4. **Behavioral Recommendations**
   - Suggests meal timing, fiber intake, or probiotic/prebiotic foods based on individual digestion patterns.

Why Gut Health Matters for Performance

- **Nutrient Absorption**: Even a perfect diet is wasted if nutrients aren't absorbed efficiently.
- **Energy Stability**: Poor gut health leads to blood sugar swings and fatigue.
- **Immune Function**: A large portion of immune activity begins in the gut.
- **Inflammation Control**: Balanced gut flora reduces systemic inflammation, supporting recovery.

Real-World Example

What Happened
A 32-year-old weightlifter followed a high-protein diet but constantly felt bloated and sluggish.

What Changed
Her AI app connected food logs with digestive symptoms and highlighted dairy protein shakes as the culprit. It suggested plant-based protein powders and increasing probiotic-rich foods like kefir and sauerkraut.

Results
Digestive discomfort disappeared, energy stabilized, and her training intensity improved noticeably.

What We Learn
Gut health isn't just about comfort — it directly influences performance and recovery.

Common Pitfalls

- **Over-Restricting Foods**: Cutting out entire groups without evidence can harm nutrient intake.
- **Chasing Quick Fixes**: Supplements without addressing underlying habits rarely solve digestion issues.

- **Ignoring Fiber Balance**: Both too little and too much fiber can create problems.
- **One-Size Advice**: Gut health is highly individual; what works for one person may harm another.

Tactical Best Practices

- **Log Symptoms Alongside Meals**: AI can only identify patterns if you track consistently.
- **Prioritize Whole Foods**: Reduce processed foods that disrupt gut flora.
- **Incorporate Prebiotics and Probiotics**: Foods like garlic, bananas, yogurt, and kimchi support gut diversity.
- **Stay Hydrated**: Digestion efficiency depends on proper fluid intake.
- **Reassess Regularly**: The gut adapts — what triggers you now may change over time.

Final Thought

Gut health is a silent driver of success in fitness and wellness. By uncovering patterns between food, symptoms, and performance, AI takes the guesswork out of digestion. With personalized insights, it empowers you to build a diet that not only fuels the body but also keeps the digestive system in balance.

Next Steps
With digestion optimized, the next step is timing. In the following section, we'll explore **Nutrient Timing for Performance** — how AI helps structure meals around training and recovery to maximize energy, endurance, and results.

Nutrient Timing for Performance

Eating the right foods is only half the equation; eating them at the right **time** can be the difference between thriving and stalling. Nutrient timing is about aligning meals and supplements with your body's activity cycles — workouts, recovery windows, and even sleep — to maximize performance and adaptation. Traditionally, this was left to guesswork or rigid bodybuilding rules. AI now makes nutrient timing practical, personalized, and dynamic.

How AI Optimizes Nutrient Timing

1. **Pre-Workout Fueling**
   - Analyzes workout intensity and duration.
   - Suggests the ideal balance of carbs (for energy) and protein (for muscle preservation).
2. **Intra-Workout Support**
   - For endurance or high-volume sessions, AI recommends hydration and electrolytes, and in some cases carb intake mid-session.
3. **Post-Workout Recovery**
   - Detects training load and recommends protein + carb windows to maximize glycogen replenishment and muscle repair.
4. **Daily Energy Management**
   - Suggests higher carb intake earlier or later depending on your glucose trends, lifestyle, and circadian rhythm.
5. **Sleep Optimization**
   - Identifies whether evening protein or magnesium-rich snacks may improve sleep quality.

Why Timing Matters

- **Maximizes Training Output**: Fueling before workouts prevents early fatigue.
- **Enhances Recovery**: Post-workout timing accelerates repair and reduces soreness.
- **Balances Energy**: Prevents midday slumps and late-night cravings.
- **Supports Hormones**: Consistent timing stabilizes insulin, cortisol, and melatonin cycles.

Real-World Example

What Happened
A 27-year-old sprinter fueled randomly throughout the day, often skipping meals before training. She felt sluggish and underperformed in workouts.

What Changed
Her AI app analyzed her training schedule and recommended pre-session carbs and post-session protein recovery meals.

Results
Her energy improved dramatically, recovery times shortened, and sprint performance hit new highs.

What We Learn
When you eat can matter just as much as what you eat — especially for performance-driven goals.

Common Pitfalls

- **Overcomplicating Timing**: Not every snack needs to be timed to the minute.
- **Ignoring Total Intake**: Timing helps, but overall calorie and macro balance matter more.

- **Carb Fear**: Skipping carbs around workouts can reduce performance and recovery.
- **Neglecting Recovery Meals**: Many underestimate how crucial post-training nutrition is.

Tactical Best Practices

- **Fuel Before Training**: Aim for a balanced carb + protein meal 1–2 hours pre-workout.
- **Don't Skip Recovery Windows**: Prioritize protein (20–40g) and carbs within 2 hours post-workout.
- **Hydrate Proactively**: Don't wait for thirst — plan water and electrolytes around activity.
- **Let AI Guide Variability**: High-intensity days may require more carbs; low-intensity days may lean toward fats.
- **Pair with Sleep Goals**: Evening snacks should support rest, not disrupt it.

Final Thought

Nutrient timing takes good nutrition and makes it **strategic.** With AI tracking workouts, recovery, and lifestyle factors, you no longer have to guess when to eat. Instead, your meals become tools — fueling performance, enhancing recovery, and supporting long-term progress.

Next Steps
Beyond timing, long-term health depends on prevention. In the next section, we'll explore **Preventing Deficiencies with Predictive Analysis**, where AI forecasts potential nutrient shortfalls before they occur and helps you stay ahead of health risks.

Preventing Deficiencies with Predictive Analysis

Nutrient deficiencies rarely appear overnight. They build slowly — often unnoticed until fatigue, poor performance, or even illness sets in. By the time symptoms surface, the body may already be under strain. Traditional approaches to detecting deficiencies rely on blood tests or waiting for symptoms, both of which are reactive.

AI changes this by using **predictive analysis**. Instead of waiting for a problem, it forecasts risks based on your diet, lifestyle, environment, and biometrics — giving you the chance to make adjustments before deficiencies ever develop.

How Predictive Analysis Works

1. **Dietary Pattern Tracking**
   - AI scans your food logs and highlights nutrients consistently under target.
   - Flags trends that may lead to long-term gaps (e.g., chronically low iron in plant-based eaters).
2. **Integration with Lifestyle Data**
   - Considers unique demands like heavy training, frequent travel, or limited sun exposure.
   - Adjusts predictions seasonally (e.g., vitamin D risk in winter months).
3. **Cross-Metric Correlation**
   - Links recovery struggles, sleep issues, or fatigue with possible micronutrient shortfalls.
4. **Forecasting Models**
   - Projects potential deficiencies weeks or months ahead and suggests early interventions.

Why Prevention Matters

- **Performance Preservation**: Keeps energy, endurance, and strength consistent.
- **Health Protection**: Prevents chronic conditions linked to long-term deficiencies.
- **Cost Efficiency**: Avoids expensive medical interventions later.
- **Peace of Mind**: Users know they're staying ahead of risks, not reacting to them.

Real-World Example

What Happened
A 36-year-old vegan athlete trained intensely but often felt tired mid-season. Bloodwork eventually showed iron deficiency.

What Changed
Her AI app analyzed her food logs, noted low iron-rich plant foods, and predicted a deficiency risk weeks earlier. It suggested lentils, spinach, and fortified cereals, plus iron supplementation if fatigue persisted.

Results
By acting early, she stabilized energy levels and avoided the full onset of anemia.

What We Learn
Predictive analysis turns nutrition from damage control into proactive health management.

Common Pitfalls

- **Assuming Perfection from AI Alone**: Forecasts are powerful but should be validated with lab work.
- **Over-Supplementation "Just in Case"**: Taking unnecessary supplements without confirmation can be harmful.

- **Ignoring Seasonal or Lifestyle Shifts**: A desk worker and an endurance athlete require different risk profiles.
- **Poor Logging Habits**: Incomplete data limits accuracy.

Tactical Best Practices

- **Log Food Consistently**: Even partial logging gives AI better insight into patterns.
- **Sync Seasonal Data**: Let AI know about lifestyle changes (e.g., travel, off-season).
- **Confirm with Bloodwork**: Validate AI predictions annually for accuracy.
- **Act Early but Conservatively**: Start with food solutions before supplementing.
- **Reassess Quarterly**: Risks shift with training cycles and lifestyle changes.

Final Thought

Preventing deficiencies isn't glamorous, but it's one of the smartest strategies for long-term health and performance. With predictive AI analysis, you stay ahead of risks instead of reacting to them, ensuring your body always has the resources it needs to adapt, recover, and thrive.

Next Steps
With nutrition fully optimized, we now move into **Chapter 10 – Long-Term Health & Lifestyle with AI**, exploring how intelligent systems extend beyond fitness goals to support sustainable health, longevity, and balanced living.

CHAPTER 10

Long-Term Health & Lifestyle with AI

Building Sustainable Habits with AI Reminders

Short-term motivation can get you started, but long-term success comes from **habits.** The small, consistent actions — like hydrating properly, hitting protein targets, or going to bed on time — are what compound into meaningful results. The challenge is that life's chaos often interrupts even the best intentions.

AI makes habit-building more sustainable by acting as an intelligent accountability partner. Unlike generic alarms or calendar reminders, AI reminders are **context-aware**: they adapt based on your behavior, schedule, and even mood, nudging you at the right time with the right message.

How AI Supports Habit Formation

1. **Contextual Nudges**
   o Instead of a fixed reminder, AI checks your readiness. Example: if your step count is low by 5 p.m., it suggests a short walk before dinner.
2. **Streak Tracking**
   o Reinforces consistency with progress streaks and micro-goals that build momentum.
3. **Adaptive Timing**
   o Learns when you're most receptive. If you often dismiss morning hydration reminders, it reschedules them later in the day.
4. **Behavioral Reinforcement**
   o Celebrates small wins (e.g., "You hit your protein target 5 days in a row!") to keep habits sticky.
5. **Goal Alignment**
   o Aligns reminders with evolving priorities. If you shift from fat loss to performance, reminders adapt accordingly.

Why This Matters

- **Consistency > Perfection**: Habits built with reminders turn occasional wins into long-term routines.
- **Reduces Mental Load**: AI tracks the details so you don't have to.
- **Personalized Support**: Reminders feel relevant instead of nagging.
- **Sustainable Change**: Builds health behaviors into your lifestyle rather than short-term fixes.

Real-World Example

What Happened
A 40-year-old professional wanted to improve sleep but frequently stayed up late working.

What Changed
Her AI platform began sending wind-down reminders tied to her recovery scores. It suggested dimming lights, reducing screen time, and logging her evening reflection.

Results
She gradually built a consistent bedtime routine, improved sleep quality, and noticed better energy during workouts.

What We Learn
Well-timed nudges can transform intentions into consistent, automated behaviors.

Common Pitfalls

- **Notification Fatigue**: Too many reminders become overwhelming.
- **Generic Messaging**: Non-personalized nudges feel easy to ignore.

- **Short-Term Engagement Only**: Reminders must evolve as habits become ingrained.
- **Over-Dependence**: True habit formation should eventually work without prompts.

Tactical Best Practices

- **Start Small**: Build one or two habits at a time to avoid overload.
- **Use AI Flexibility**: Allow the system to adjust timing if you keep dismissing reminders.
- **Pair Reminders With Triggers**: Example: "After lunch, take a 10-minute walk."
- **Celebrate Streaks**: Use gamified streak tracking to reinforce behavior.
- **Transition to Autonomy**: Over time, scale back reminders once the habit sticks.

Final Thought

Sustainable health isn't built in big lcaps — it's built in daily choices. AI reminders ensure those choices happen consistently by nudging you at the right time with the right action. Over time, these nudges transform into habits, and habits evolve into lifestyle.

Next Steps
With habits forming, the next step is **AI for Behavior Tracking and Pattern Recognition** — how intelligent systems spot trends in your actions, identify weak points, and guide smarter long-term decision-making.

AI for Behavior Tracking and Pattern Recognition

One of the biggest challenges in building a healthy lifestyle is **self-awareness.** Many people don't realize how often they skip workouts, overeat late at night, or sacrifice sleep until the negative effects pile up. Behavior tracking powered by AI brings these blind spots into the open, helping you see patterns that are otherwise invisible.

By monitoring your choices over weeks and months, AI doesn't just count what you do — it interprets your behaviors, detects trends, and shows you where small shifts can have the biggest impact.

How AI Tracks and Recognizes Patterns

1. **Workout Consistency**
   o Identifies missed sessions or declining intensity across training cycles.
2. **Nutrition Habits**
   o Detects recurring late-night snacking, weekend overeating, or protein shortfalls.
3. **Sleep & Recovery Behaviors**
   o Recognizes when poor sleep aligns with stress spikes or skipped workouts.
4. **Lifestyle Routines**
   o Spots correlations like increased alcohol use during high-stress weeks or lower activity during colder months.
5. **Emotional Triggers**
   o Links mood logs and adherence data to highlight emotional eating or stress-driven lapses.

Why Pattern Recognition Matters

- **Early Intervention**: AI flags patterns before they spiral into major setbacks.
- **Personal Insight**: Helps you understand not just *what* you do, but *why.*
- **Better Goal Alignment**: Ensures daily actions reflect long-term health objectives.
- **Sustainable Lifestyle**: Identifies where small, realistic changes beat dramatic overhauls.

Real-World Example

What Happened
A 35-year-old teacher consistently logged workouts but couldn't understand why fat loss stalled.

What Changed
Her AI system detected a recurring pattern: late-night calorie spikes after stressful days, which offset her otherwise consistent nutrition.

Results
With this awareness, she introduced healthier evening rituals and adjusted her dinner macros. Within weeks, progress resumed.

What We Learn
Patterns matter more than isolated choices — AI makes them visible and actionable.

Common Pitfalls

- **Data Blindness**: Collecting metrics without analyzing them leads nowhere.
- **Over-Focus on Small Deviations**: One skipped workout isn't a trend — AI looks for repeated behaviors.
- **Resistance to Feedback**: Some users ignore patterns that challenge their self-perception.
- **Neglecting Emotional Context**: Data without self-reflection misses the "why" behind habits.

Tactical Best Practices

- **Log Honestly**: AI accuracy depends on complete, truthful inputs.
- **Review Weekly Reports**: Look for 2–3 recurring habits, not daily fluctuations.
- **Act on Small Adjustments**: Address weak points with simple fixes, not massive overhauls.

- **Pair Data With Reflection**: Note how you felt on days patterns repeated.
- **Stay Patient**: Long-term trends are more valuable than daily noise.

Final Thought

Behavior tracking and pattern recognition help you see yourself clearly. Instead of reacting to every slip, AI highlights the underlying trends that shape long-term outcomes. With this awareness, you can make smarter, more sustainable adjustments — building a lifestyle that works for you, not against you.

Next Steps
Awareness is powerful, but prevention is better. In the next section, we'll explore **Preventing Relapse with Proactive Alerts** — how AI systems anticipate setbacks and send timely nudges to keep you from slipping back into old habits.

Preventing Relapse with Proactive Alerts

Making progress is hard, but keeping it is often harder. Many people achieve initial success, only to relapse into old habits when life gets stressful, busy, or unpredictable. Relapses rarely happen overnight — they're the result of small lapses that accumulate over time.

AI reduces relapse risk by issuing **proactive alerts**: timely nudges based on your behavior, environment, and biometric signals. Instead of waiting for setbacks to unfold, AI helps you catch warning signs early, steering you back on track before momentum is lost.

How AI Prevents Relapse

1. **Consistency Alerts**
   - Detects missed workouts, reduced step counts, or logging gaps and prompts a gentle reminder.

2. **Nutritional Slippage**
   o Flags repeated late-night snacking, weekend calorie surges, or skipped protein targets.
3. **Recovery Red Flags**
   o Warns when sleep quality drops or stress scores climb for multiple days in a row.
4. **Seasonal & Situational Risks**
   o Predicts high-risk relapse windows such as holidays, travel, or busy work cycles.
5. **Personalized Nudges**
   o Instead of generic messages, AI offers actionable alternatives (e.g., "Missed your long run? Here's a 20-minute session to keep streak alive.").

Why Proactive Alerts Matter

- **Stops Small Slips From Snowballing**: A missed workout is just a blip — unless it becomes a pattern.
- **Boosts Accountability**: Keeps you engaged without relying solely on willpower.
- **Reduces Stress of Setbacks**: Reframes missed habits as opportunities to adjust, not failures.
- **Maintains Long-Term Progress**: Prevents cycles of start-stop dieting or inconsistent training.

Real-World Example

What Happened
A 42-year-old father lost 25 pounds but often regained weight during busy work travel.

What Changed
His AI app tracked patterns of skipped workouts and late-night meals during trips. Before his next travel week, it issued proactive alerts: prepping portable meals, scheduling short hotel workouts, and setting reminders for hydration.

Results
He completed the trip without relapse, maintained his weight loss, and felt in control instead of reactive.

What We Learn
Relapse prevention isn't about perfection — it's about timely interventions that keep momentum alive.

Common Pitfalls

- **Alert Fatigue**: Too many reminders can feel overwhelming or easy to ignore.
- **Generic Messages**: Alerts must be personalized and context-specific to be effective.
- **Ignoring Human Context**: Some setbacks (family emergencies, illness) require flexibility, not just nudges.
- **All-or-Nothing Mindset**: Users may treat one relapse as total failure without AI reframing.

Tactical Best Practices

- **Set Alert Thresholds**: Decide how many missed workouts or poor sleep nights trigger notifications.
- **Keep Alerts Actionable**: Pair nudges with practical next steps, not just warnings.
- **Balance Flexibility and Structure**: Use alerts to guide, not guilt-trip.
- **Review Weekly**: Use alerts as learning opportunities to refine future strategies.
- **Pair With Reflection**: Log how you handled alerts to build resilience.

Final Thought

Relapse isn't inevitable. With proactive AI alerts, small lapses become opportunities for adjustment rather than slippery slopes into old habits. By anticipating risk and guiding you with timely, personalized nudges, AI transforms the fight against relapse into a system of steady, sustainable growth.

Next Steps
With relapse prevention in place, the next section will cover **AI-Assisted Lifestyle Balance (Workouts, Diet, Rest)** — how intelligent systems orchestrate the three pillars of health into a harmonious rhythm that supports both performance and longevity.

AI-Assisted Lifestyle Balance (Workouts, Diet, Rest)

Fitness success doesn't come from exercise alone, or diet alone, or even perfect recovery. It comes from **balance** — the ongoing alignment of training, nutrition, and rest with your life's demands. Too often, people push too hard in one area and neglect the others: dieting without strength, training without sleep, or resting without movement. The result? Burnout, plateaus, or short-lived results.

AI excels at balancing these pillars. By analyzing your biometric data, schedule, and habits, it acts like a conductor — ensuring workouts, diet, and recovery work in harmony instead of conflict.

How AI Creates Balance

1. **Workouts**
   o Adjusts training load based on recovery and energy levels.
   o Ensures intensity matches your readiness to prevent overtraining.

2. **Diet**
   - ○ Aligns nutrition with your activity cycle (higher carbs on training days, balanced macros on recovery days).
   - ○ Flags when your calorie intake mismatches your training volume.
3. **Rest & Recovery**
   - ○ Tracks sleep and stress to recommend rest days or lighter workouts.
   - ○ Suggests mindfulness or active recovery when fatigue is detected.
4. **Integration Across Systems**
   - ○ Combines inputs from wearables, nutrition logs, and workout apps into one cohesive plan.
   - ○ Provides daily and weekly balance scores showing how well the three pillars align.

Why Balance Matters

- **Consistency**: Balanced plans are more sustainable than extreme approaches.
- **Adaptability**: Keeps you on track when life throws curveballs.
- **Injury Prevention**: Reduces the risk of burnout or overuse.
- **Optimal Results**: Progress comes faster when all three pillars support one another.

Real-World Example

What Happened
A 33-year-old entrepreneur trained intensely five days a week while cutting calories aggressively. He quickly burned out, lost muscle mass, and stalled fat loss.

What Changed
His AI platform flagged poor recovery and nutrient mismatches. It restructured his plan: fewer high-intensity sessions, added recovery days, and better carb timing around workouts.

Results
Energy levels rebounded, he began gaining lean muscle, and fat loss resumed steadily.

What We Learn
Fitness progress isn't about extremes — it's about balance.

Common Pitfalls

- **Overvaluing One Pillar**: Training harder won't fix a poor diet or lack of sleep.
- **Ignoring Recovery**: Many treat rest as optional when it's foundational.
- **Short-Term Focus**: Unsustainable crash diets or training streaks cause long-term setbacks.
- **Fragmented Tracking**: Using separate apps without integration creates blind spots.

Tactical Best Practices

- **Track All Three Pillars Together**: Let AI integrate training, nutrition, and rest for a full picture.
- **Prioritize Recovery**: Treat sleep and stress as seriously as workouts.
- **Align Food With Activity**: Match carbs, protein, and calories to training vs. rest days.
- **Review Balance Scores Weekly**: Use AI summaries to adjust before burnout hits.
- **Stay Flexible**: Balance doesn't mean rigid perfection — it means consistent alignment.

Final Thought

Sustainable health is a three-legged stool: workouts, diet, and rest. Remove one, and the system collapses. AI's unique strength is its ability to weave these elements together, keeping you aligned and adaptive no matter what life throws at you.

Next Steps

Balance is the foundation of long-term success, but growth doesn't stop there. In the next section, we'll explore **Lifelong Learning: How AI Evolves With You** — showing how intelligent systems adapt over decades, growing alongside your needs, goals, and lifestyle.

Lifelong Learning: How AI Evolves With You

Health is not static. The goals you set at 25 — chasing athletic performance or fat loss — are rarely the same ones you prioritize at 45, 60, or beyond. Life stages bring new challenges: shifting metabolisms, injuries, careers, family responsibilities, and evolving definitions of "fitness." Too often, people cling to outdated routines that no longer match their bodies or lifestyles.

AI solves this by being a **lifelong learner.** Unlike rigid programs or fad diets, AI platforms evolve with you. They adapt as your data, goals, and circumstances change — ensuring your health strategy remains relevant not just for months, but for decades.

How AI Learns Over Time

1. **Cumulative Data Collection**
   - Builds a long-term profile of your habits, performance, and health markers.
   - Learns your unique responses to training, diet, and recovery.
2. **Adaptive Goal Shifts**
   - Transitions from fat loss to maintenance, from performance to longevity, as your life priorities shift.
3. **Context Awareness**
   - Recognizes major lifestyle changes (new job, parenthood, travel, aging) and adjusts recommendations accordingly.

4. **Predictive Adjustments**
   - Anticipates when plateaus or setbacks are likely, based on your history, and suggests preventive changes.
5. **Continuous Refinement**
   - Uses each success or failure as feedback to fine-tune your next strategy.

Why Lifelong AI Guidance Matters

- **Relevance**: Your program never becomes outdated.
- **Sustainability**: Eliminates the cycle of starting over every few years.
- **Confidence**: Provides clarity during life transitions when many lose direction.
- **Holistic Support**: Adapts to physical, emotional, and lifestyle changes over decades.

Real-World Example

What Happened
A 27-year-old began using an AI platform to lose weight. Over 15 years, his life changed dramatically — career growth, children, injuries, and eventually shifting focus toward longevity.

What Changed
His AI system adapted each phase: weight loss to strength building, strength to injury-friendly programming, and later to cardiovascular and mobility support. Nutrition shifted from aggressive dieting to sustainable energy balance.

Results
Instead of yo-yo cycles, he maintained consistent health across decades with plans that always matched his reality.

What We Learn
The real value of AI isn't just short-term optimization — it's lifelong evolution.

Common Pitfalls

- **Treating AI as Static**: Not updating goals or life changes reduces its effectiveness.
- **Neglecting Long-Term Data**: Inconsistent logging weakens the AI's ability to adapt.
- **Focusing Only on Short-Term Wins**: Forgetting that health strategies must last decades, not weeks.
- **Ignoring Shifts in Priorities**: Goals like mobility and recovery become as important as aesthetics over time.

Tactical Best Practices

- **Update Goals Regularly**: Revisit your targets quarterly to keep AI aligned.
- **Log Life Changes**: Inform AI about stress, injuries, or new routines for accurate recommendations.
- **Think in Decades**: Use AI not just for the next 30 days but for sustainable growth over years.
- **Review Long-Term Reports**: Look for yearly and decade-level trends in addition to weekly results.
- **Embrace Evolution**: Accept that your body and priorities will change — and let AI guide the transition.

Final Thought

Health isn't a sprint — it's a lifelong journey. AI acts as a companion that grows with you, learning your body's rhythms and adapting to each new stage of life. With its continuous evolution, it ensures you never outgrow your health strategy, no matter where life takes you.

Next Steps
With lifelong adaptability established, the next section dives deeper into the future: **AI Insights into Aging and Longevity Support** — how intelligent systems can optimize not just performance today, but vitality and independence for the decades ahead.

AI Insights into Aging and Longevity Support

Longevity is no longer just about living longer — it's about living **better.** Modern health science emphasizes not only lifespan but "healthspan": the number of years you remain active, independent, and vibrant. As people age, the focus naturally shifts from peak performance and aesthetics to joint health, cognitive resilience, disease prevention, and overall vitality.

AI is emerging as a powerful ally in this space. By continuously analyzing health markers, predicting risks, and personalizing routines, it provides practical insights into how to age gracefully — turning longevity from an abstract concept into actionable, daily habits.

How AI Supports Aging and Longevity

1. **Early Risk Detection**
   o Identifies subtle patterns in biometrics (e.g., declining HRV, rising resting heart rate) that may signal long-term cardiovascular or metabolic risks.
2. **Mobility & Joint Health Monitoring**
   o Tracks movement quality through wearables or video analysis, detecting changes in flexibility, balance, or stability before they become functional issues.
3. **Cognitive Support**
   o Monitors sleep quality, stress, and activity levels tied to brain health.
   o Suggests habits that promote neuroplasticity, such as new skill learning or mindfulness.
4. **Nutritional Adjustments**
   o Accounts for age-related changes in metabolism and nutrient absorption.
   o Flags higher needs for protein, vitamin D, calcium, and omega-3s to maintain bone and muscle health.

5. **Longevity Programming**
     o Designs workouts prioritizing strength, mobility, and
       cardiovascular efficiency — proven anchors of
       healthy aging.

Why This Matters

- **Independence**: Strong muscles, flexible joints, and balance
  reduce fall risks and prolong autonomy.
- **Disease Prevention**: Data-driven monitoring helps mitigate
  risks of diabetes, heart disease, and osteoporosis.
- **Quality of Life**: Supports energy, mental sharpness, and
  physical confidence well into later decades.
- **Personalization**: Aging looks different for everyone — AI
  adjusts to *your* trajectory.

Real-World Example

What Happened
A 58-year-old executive wanted to maintain vitality but struggled
with energy and joint stiffness.

What Changed
His AI health platform integrated his training data, sleep patterns,
and nutrition logs. It flagged low protein intake, suggested mobility-
focused workouts, and encouraged daily walks instead of more high-
impact cardio.

Results
His energy improved, joint discomfort decreased, and he built a
routine that felt sustainable.

What We Learn
Longevity support doesn't come from extreme programs — it comes
from consistent, data-informed adjustments.

Common Pitfalls

- **Chasing Youthful Performance**: Ignoring shifting priorities leads to burnout or injury.
- **One-Size-Fits-All Aging Advice**: Generic longevity "hacks" ignore individual data.
- **Overlooking Recovery**: Sleep and stress management become more crucial with age.
- **Focusing Only on Lifespan**: Living longer without maintaining function misses the point.

Tactical Best Practices

- **Track Functional Metrics**: Strength, balance, and flexibility matter as much as weight.
- **Reassess Nutrition Regularly**: Age alters absorption — adjust protein, calcium, and vitamin D intake accordingly.
- **Emphasize Mobility Work**: Daily flexibility and stability drills maintain independence.
- **Use AI Risk Forecasts**: Treat flagged risks as opportunities for prevention, not fear.
- **Think in Decades, Not Weeks**: Adopt routines that support vitality for the long haul.

Final Thought

Aging well isn't about resisting time — it's about working with it intelligently. AI provides the tools to track, predict, and optimize the factors that truly influence healthspan. By guiding daily choices around movement, nutrition, and recovery, it helps you add not just years to life, but life to your years.

Next Steps
With longevity insights covered, we now turn to a critical dimension of this journey: **Chapter 11 – Ethics, Privacy & Human Control**, where we'll examine the responsibilities, risks, and safeguards necessary when entrusting personal health data to AI systems.

CHAPTER 11

Ethics, Privacy & Human Control

The Risks of Overreliance on AI in Health

AI has transformed the way we track, analyze, and improve health. But with its growing influence comes an important caveat: **no algorithm can replace human judgment, context, or responsibility.** Overreliance on AI in fitness and wellness carries risks that can undermine both safety and autonomy if left unchecked.

AI is a tool — not a substitute for critical thinking, professional medical care, or personal accountability. Recognizing its limitations ensures that technology enhances health rather than dictating it.

Key Risks of Overreliance

1. **Loss of Autonomy**
   o   Blindly following AI recommendations can erode personal intuition about how your body feels.
2. **Algorithmic Gaps**
   o   AI relies on the quality of its data. If inputs are incomplete, biased, or incorrect, outputs may misguide.
3. **Ignoring Human Context**
   o   AI can't fully account for emotional stress, personal values, or sudden life changes.
4. **Safety Concerns**
   o   Automated adjustments to diet, training, or supplementation without medical oversight may create unintended health risks.
5. **Dependency Risk**
   o   Users may struggle to self-manage without technology, losing confidence in their ability to make decisions.

Real-World Example

What Happened
A 29-year-old relied exclusively on an AI app to design workouts and monitor diet. When the app flagged him as "recovered," he pushed through a session despite feeling exhausted.

What Changed
He strained his lower back, leading to weeks of reduced activity. His doctor noted that listening to his own fatigue cues might have prevented the injury.

Results
He adjusted his approach — using AI for structure, but also checking in with his body and occasionally seeking professional advice.

What We Learn
AI guidance is valuable, but ignoring human intuition and context can lead to setbacks.

Common Pitfalls

- **Data Blindness**: Treating AI outputs as "truth" instead of tools for decision-making.
- **One-Size Assumptions**: Believing algorithms can account for every unique health variable.
- **Skipping Professional Input**: Avoiding doctors or coaches in favor of app-based advice.
- **Emotional Detachment**: Reducing health to numbers instead of considering the full human experience.

Tactical Best Practices

- **Balance AI With Intuition**: Use technology to guide, not dictate, decisions.
- **Validate Major Changes**: Consult professionals before adopting extreme AI-driven adjustments.

- **Use AI as a Co-Pilot**: Let it handle tracking and analysis while you make final calls.
- **Stay Critical**: Question recommendations and verify data sources when in doubt.
- **Develop Self-Awareness**: Regularly reflect on how your body feels beyond what AI reports.

Final Thought

AI is a powerful amplifier of health, but it must remain a **partner, not a master.** Overreliance risks undermining the very self-awareness and autonomy that make health sustainable. The best outcomes come when AI supports human judgment, not replaces it.

Next Steps
One of the biggest ethical concerns tied to AI in health is privacy. In the next section, we'll explore **Protecting Personal Health Data** — how to safeguard sensitive information while benefiting from the power of intelligent systems.

Protecting Personal Health Data

AI's ability to personalize health strategies relies on data — and lots of it. From sleep cycles and heart rate variability to nutrition logs and even microbiome samples, these insights fuel AI's recommendations. But the same data that drives progress is also deeply personal, sensitive, and potentially vulnerable. If mishandled, health data can be misused by companies, insurers, or even malicious actors.

Protecting personal health data is not just a technical necessity — it's an ethical responsibility. To benefit from AI while safeguarding trust, users and providers alike must prioritize privacy, security, and informed consent.

Risks of Poor Data Protection

1. **Unauthorized Access**
   o Breaches can expose sensitive medical or lifestyle details.
2. **Commercial Exploitation**
   o Data may be sold to advertisers or third parties without transparent consent.
3. **Insurance or Employment Bias**
   o Misuse of health metrics could influence premiums or workplace decisions.
4. **Loss of Control**
   o Users may not know how their information is stored, shared, or deleted.

How to Safeguard Your Health Data

- **Choose Trusted Platforms**: Work with AI providers that clearly state how data is used and protected.
- **Check Encryption Standards**: Ensure platforms use end-to-end encryption for storage and transmission.
- **Limit Permissions**: Only share data necessary for the app's function.
- **Review Privacy Policies**: Look for transparency around third-party sharing.
- **Exercise Data Rights**: Request data deletion or export when switching services.

Real-World Example

What Happened
A fitness enthusiast used a free AI nutrition tracker that quietly sold her data to advertisers. Soon, she was targeted with aggressive supplement ads tailored to her logged deficiencies.

What Changed
After switching to a paid platform with transparent privacy policies, she regained confidence that her information was being used ethically.

Results
She continued benefiting from AI insights without compromising her privacy.

What We Learn
"Free" apps often come at the cost of your personal data. Transparency matters more than price.

Common Pitfalls

- **Ignoring Terms & Conditions**: Many users skip reading how their data is used.
- **Assuming All Apps Are Equal**: Privacy standards vary widely between platforms.
- **Over-Sharing**: Granting unnecessary device or account permissions.
- **Neglecting Updates**: Outdated apps can be more vulnerable to breaches.

Tactical Best Practices

- **Vet Before You Download**: Research company history and reputation.
- **Pay for Privacy**: Subscription-based models are less likely to monetize data.
- **Use Strong Authentication**: Enable two-factor authentication for accounts.
- **Audit Permissions Quarterly**: Revoke access apps no longer need.
- **Own Your Data**: Prioritize platforms that let you export and control your information.

Final Thought

Your health data is one of your most valuable assets. Protecting it means protecting your future — not just from hackers, but from misuse by businesses or institutions. With the right precautions, AI can remain a tool for empowerment rather than a source of vulnerability.

Next Steps
Beyond security, balance is also about decision-making. In the next section, we'll discuss **The Role of Human Intuition Alongside AI** — how to blend data-driven insights with your own self-awareness for the best long-term outcomes.

The Role of Human Intuition Alongside AI

AI excels at identifying patterns, predicting outcomes, and guiding decisions with data. But no algorithm — no matter how advanced — can replace the lived experience of being human. Your body communicates through signals: hunger, fatigue, soreness, stress, and emotion. These cues can't always be quantified, but they are essential for long-term health.

The challenge lies in striking a balance: using AI for clarity and structure without silencing your own intuition. When data-driven insights work alongside human awareness, the result is a healthier, more sustainable approach.

Why Intuition Matters

1. **Immediate Feedback**
    o   AI processes historical and real-time data, but only you feel the subtle differences between "tired" and "exhausted."

2. **Emotional Context**
   - o Stress, joy, or grief all affect how you respond to food and exercise. AI may not fully account for these nuances.
3. **Adaptability in the Moment**
   - o Sometimes the best decision isn't what the app suggests — it's taking an unplanned rest day or sharing dessert with friends.
4. **Preventing Overreliance**
   - o Intuition ensures you don't become dependent on technology to make every choice.

Real-World Example

What Happened
A 30-year-old followed her AI training app religiously. Despite recurring knee pain, she continued workouts because her readiness score appeared "green."

What Changed
She decided to listen to her own signals, took a week of modified training, and sought physiotherapy.

Results
Her knee recovered, and she returned to training stronger.

What We Learn
AI is a guide, not an authority. Human intuition ensures safe, context-driven decisions.

Common Pitfalls

- **Data Obsession**: Ignoring how you feel in favor of what the numbers say.
- **Distrust of Self**: Believing you can't make good choices without AI guidance.

- **Perfectionism**: Following recommendations so rigidly that flexibility disappears.
- **Ignoring Emotional Health**: Reducing wellness to numbers while neglecting joy or social connection.

Tactical Best Practices

- **Use Data as a Compass, Not a Map**: Let AI guide direction, but let intuition choose the route.
- **Check In Daily**: Ask yourself: "How do I feel?" before looking at metrics.
- **Build Flex Days**: Allow untracked meals or unstructured workouts to maintain balance.
- **Learn From Discomfort**: Use pain, fatigue, or cravings as signals, not failures.
- **Blend Logic and Feeling**: Combine AI trends with self-awareness to make holistic choices.

Final Thought

Human intuition provides the emotional and physical context that AI cannot. When paired together, they form a powerful partnership: data provides clarity, intuition provides wisdom. Trusting both ensures progress is not only measurable but meaningful.

Next Steps
When tracking goes too far, it risks harm. In the next section, we'll explore **Avoiding Disordered Eating Amplified by Tracking Apps** — how to use AI responsibly without turning health tools into unhealthy obsessions.

Avoiding Disordered Eating Amplified by Tracking Apps

Nutrition tracking apps and AI diet planners can be powerful tools for awareness and accountability. But when every calorie, macro, or bite of food becomes a number to be judged, the line between healthy monitoring and unhealthy obsession can blur. For some, the constant measurement can trigger or worsen **disordered eating behaviors** — such as guilt around food, restrictive patterns, or compulsive logging.

AI systems must be designed and used in a way that **supports health without fueling obsession.** Recognizing these risks helps ensure that tracking apps remain tools for empowerment, not sources of harm.

How Tracking Can Go Wrong

1. **Rigid Perfectionism**
   - Feeling compelled to hit calorie or macro targets exactly every day, creating guilt when falling short.
2. **Over-Focus on Numbers**
   - Valuing numbers (calories, grams, streaks) over body signals like hunger or fullness.
3. **Guilt & Shame Cycles**
   - Punishing oneself after "bad" days rather than seeing nutrition in the bigger picture.
4. **Loss of Flexibility**
   - Avoiding social meals or treats because they're harder to log accurately.

Safeguards AI Can Provide

- **Healthy Range Targets**
  - Instead of exact numbers, AI can recommend ranges (e.g., 90–110g protein) to reduce rigidity.
- **Positive Reinforcement**
  - Focuses on consistency and trends, not punishing small deviations.
- **Intuitive Eating Integration**
  - Encourages reflection on hunger, satiety, and enjoyment alongside calorie counts.
- **Break Features**
  - Suggests tracking breaks when adherence becomes compulsive.

- **Mental Health Flags**
  - Detects obsessive logging patterns and nudges users toward professional support if needed.

Real-World Example

What Happened
A 25-year-old started with a calorie-tracking app for fat loss. Within months, she became anxious about going out to eat and felt guilty for exceeding her targets by even 50 calories.

What Changed
Her AI-based platform shifted her from strict daily goals to weekly trend targets. It added prompts asking, "How did this meal make you feel?" rather than only logging numbers.

Results
Her relationship with food improved, she regained social flexibility, and she continued progressing toward her goals without anxiety.

What We Learn
Health tracking must serve the person — not dominate their life.

Common Pitfalls

- **All-or-Nothing Thinking**: Treating missed targets as failure.
- **Ignoring Mental Health**: Overlooking how tracking affects mood and stress.
- **Treating Food as Only Numbers**: Forgetting food also provides culture, connection, and enjoyment.
- **Neglecting Professional Help**: Not seeking guidance when disordered behaviors emerge.

Tactical Best Practices

- **Focus on Trends, Not Perfection**: Use AI to spot weekly or monthly progress, not daily "success" or "failure."

- **Use Flexible Targets**: Accept ranges instead of rigid numbers.
- **Check Emotional Impact**: Reflect regularly: "Is tracking helping me, or stressing me?"
- **Take Breaks**: Allow days or meals without logging to maintain balance.
- **Know When to Seek Support**: If tracking creates guilt, anxiety, or compulsion, pause and consult a professional.

Final Thought

AI can help people eat smarter, but if misused, it can also amplify unhealthy food relationships. The solution isn't abandoning tracking — it's designing and using systems that encourage **flexibility, balance, and self-awareness.** The healthiest diet is one that nourishes both body and mind.

Next Steps
Beyond eating behaviors, another ethical dimension remains: **Who Owns Your Fitness Data?** In the next section, we'll examine the critical question of data ownership, control, and the power dynamics between users and the companies that collect their health information.

Who Owns Your Fitness Data?

Every step counted, calorie logged, and heartbeat measured generates data. But once that information leaves your device and enters the cloud, an important question arises: **who actually owns it?** Many users assume their health data belongs to them. In reality, terms of service agreements often grant companies the right to store, analyze, and even sell it.

This issue goes beyond privacy — it's about **control and trust.** If your health data drives AI insights that shape your habits, then ownership determines whether you remain the beneficiary, or whether your information becomes a commodity for others.

The Current Landscape

1. **User-Generated Data**
   - Technically created by you (steps, logs, biometrics) but often stored and controlled by companies.
2. **Corporate Ownership Models**
   - Many fitness apps claim broad rights to use and monetize data for research, advertising, or partnerships.
3. **Limited User Control**
   - Exporting or deleting data can be difficult, if not impossible, depending on the platform.
4. **Legal Gray Zones**
   - Unlike medical records (covered by healthcare regulations like HIPAA in the U.S.), fitness data from wearables or apps often lacks strong protections.

Why Ownership Matters

- **Privacy**: Without clear rights, your health profile may be shared without consent.
- **Monetization**: Companies can profit from your behaviors while you gain no benefit.
- **Transparency**: Ownership determines whether you know how data is being used.
- **Future Leverage**: Your lifelong data trail may one day influence insurance, employment, or access to services.

Real-World Example

What Happened
A popular wearable brand partnered with insurance companies, offering discounts for users who shared activity data. While marketed as a perk, users had little say in how long their data was stored or how else it might be used.

What Changed

Some users realized they had effectively "sold" their privacy for a short-term incentive. Opting out meant losing access to certain features of the device they had already purchased.

Results

Consumer watchdogs began calling for stronger protections and clearer ownership policies.

What We Learn

Convenience often hides hidden costs — your data may be more valuable to others than to you.

Common Pitfalls

- **Not Reading Agreements**: Most users accept terms without understanding them.
- **Assuming Portability**: Believing you can easily transfer your data between apps.
- **Trading Data for Discounts**: Underestimating long-term implications of short-tcrm pcrks.
- **Confusing Access with Ownership**: Being able to *see* your data doesn't mean you control it.

Tactical Best Practices

- **Ask Questions First**: Before using an app, check who retains ownership of your data.
- **Choose Transparent Platforms**: Favor companies that let you export or delete data easily.
- **Avoid Data-for-Discount Traps**: Consider whether incentives are worth your privacy.
- **Back Up Locally**: Store important metrics offline or in your own secure cloud.
- **Push for Policy Change**: Support platforms and regulations that prioritize user ownership.

Final Thought

Fitness data isn't just numbers — it's a digital blueprint of your health. Until ownership rights become standardized, users must remain vigilant. True empowerment means not only benefiting from AI insights but also knowing that your data ultimately belongs to you.

Next Steps
Ownership leads naturally into policy. In the next section, we'll explore **The Future of Regulation in AI Health Apps**, examining how governments and institutions are beginning to address the ethical and legal gaps in this rapidly growing field.

The Future of Regulation in AI Health Apps

AI health apps exist in a regulatory gray zone. While medical devices and clinical data are tightly regulated, most consumer health tools — step counters, workout apps, meal planners, and even advanced AI-driven platforms — fall outside traditional oversight. This creates innovation opportunities but also risks: misuse of sensitive data, inaccurate recommendations, and lack of accountability when things go wrong.

The future will require **clearer, stronger regulation** to balance innovation with protection. Governments, health institutions, and consumer advocacy groups are already beginning to shape how AI health apps will be governed in the coming years.

Emerging Regulatory Trends

1. **Data Privacy Laws**
   o Frameworks like GDPR (Europe) and CCPA (California) are setting global standards for user consent, transparency, and data rights.
2. **Medical-Grade Standards**
   o As AI apps blur the line between fitness and medicine, some will face stricter certification — especially if they diagnose or prescribe.
3. **Transparency Requirements**
   o Future regulations may force companies to explain how AI models generate recommendations.
4. **Portability and Ownership Rights**
   o Laws may increasingly require apps to allow easy export, deletion, or transfer of personal data.
5. **Algorithmic Accountability**
   o Pressure is growing for audits to ensure AI systems are fair, accurate, and free from bias.

Why Regulation Matters

- **User Safety**: Ensures recommendations don't cross into dangerous or misleading territory.
- **Privacy Protection**: Limits data exploitation by corporations.
- **Trust Building**: Clear rules make users more confident in adopting AI tools.
- **Level Playing Field**: Holds all app providers to the same ethical standards.

Real-World Example

What Happened
Several years ago, a fertility-tracking app was found to share user data with third-party advertisers without disclosure. The backlash sparked investigations and fines under GDPR.

What Changed

The incident accelerated calls for transparency and stricter oversight in consumer health apps.

Results

Companies began revising privacy policies, while regulators pushed for clearer boundaries between consumer convenience tools and medical devices.

What We Learn

Regulation often follows scandal — but proactive protections can prevent harm before it happens.

Common Pitfalls

- **Over-Regulation Fears**: Some worry too much oversight may stifle innovation.
- **Patchwork Laws**: Rules differ by country or state, creating confusion.
- **Reactive Policy**: Regulations often lag behind technology advancements.
- **Corporate Loopholes**: Companies may exploit vague legal definitions to avoid compliance.

Tactical Best Practices for Users

- **Stay Informed**: Watch how local laws evolve around health data and AI tools.
- **Favor Transparent Platforms**: Choose apps that already comply with strict privacy standards.
- **Control Your Data**: Regularly export and back up important metrics.
- **Advocate for Ethical AI**: Support companies and policies that put user safety first.
- **Expect Change**: Regulations will evolve — be ready to reassess your platforms as new standards arrive.

Final Thought

The future of AI in health isn't just about smarter algorithms — it's about smarter safeguards. Regulation will be essential in ensuring that innovation improves lives without compromising rights. For users, this means greater trust, safety, and empowerment in choosing the tools that shape their health journey.

Next Steps
With ethics and governance addressed, we now turn to the horizon. In the next chapter — **Chapter 12: The Future of AI in Fitness & Nutrition** — we'll explore upcoming technologies, trends, and possibilities that will redefine how people train, eat, and live in the decades ahead.

CHAPTER 12

The Future of AI in Fitness & Nutrition

Predictive Disease Prevention Through AI

For decades, health care has been reactive: treating disease after it appears. The next era of fitness and nutrition will flip that model. With the power of AI, prevention can become **predictive** — identifying risks long before symptoms develop and guiding daily choices that reduce the likelihood of chronic conditions.

By analyzing patterns across genetics, biometrics, lifestyle, and nutrition, AI doesn't just tell you how to get fit — it helps forecast health risks such as diabetes, cardiovascular disease, or osteoporosis. This allows individuals to act early, making lifestyle shifts that prevent illness rather than waiting for medical crises.

How Predictive Prevention Works

1. **Longitudinal Data Analysis**
   - AI tracks long-term trends in weight, activity, blood pressure, HRV, sleep, and diet.
   - Subtle shifts can indicate early markers of metabolic syndrome or cardiovascular strain.
2. **Risk Modeling**
   - Combines personal history with population-level data to estimate probabilities of future disease.
3. **Lifestyle Interventions**
   - Offers targeted nutrition, training, and recovery strategies to offset identified risks.
4. **Continuous Monitoring**
   - Wearables and health apps feed data in real time, allowing AI to detect early warning signals.
5. **Integration With Medical Systems**
   - In future models, AI may sync directly with healthcare providers, supporting preventive medicine.

Why It Matters

- **Proactive Health**: Prevents disease instead of managing it later.
- **Cost Savings**: Reduces medical expenses by addressing risks early.
- **Personal Empowerment**: Puts actionable tools in the hands of individuals.
- **Longevity Support**: Enhances healthspan by reducing age-related disease onset.

Real-World Example

What Happened
A 41-year-old with a family history of diabetes used an AI platform linked to his wearable and food logs.

What Changed
The system flagged rising fasting glucose levels and a pattern of late-night high-carb eating. It recommended more balanced meals earlier in the day, moderate resistance training, and improved sleep hygiene.

Results
Within six months, his glucose markers stabilized, reducing his long-term diabetes risk.

What We Learn
Predictive insights, paired with small daily actions, can rewrite family health legacies.

Common Pitfalls

- **False Security**: Assuming AI forecasts are guarantees rather than probabilities.
- **Neglecting Professional Oversight**: Skipping medical checkups because AI "says you're fine."

- **Data Gaps**: Incomplete tracking can weaken predictions.
- **Overwhelm From Alerts**: Too many risk notifications may cause anxiety or disengagement.

Tactical Best Practices

- **Pair With Medical Testing**: Use AI forecasts alongside regular checkups and bloodwork.
- **Act Early**: Don't wait for symptoms; address flagged risks proactively.
- **Focus on Lifestyle Levers**: Nutrition, activity, stress, and sleep are modifiable risk factors.
- **Track Consistently**: Reliable input equals more accurate predictions.
- **Use AI as a Guide, Not a Diagnosis**: Treat outputs as insights, not absolute truths.

Final Thought

Predictive prevention marks a paradigm shift: from waiting for illness to actively building a future of resilience. With AI guiding daily choices based on risk modeling, individuals can extend not just their years of life, but the quality of those years.

Next Steps
One of the most promising frontiers of this predictive future is the fusion of **AI + DNA testing for hyper-personalized nutrition** — where your genetic blueprint shapes the most precise diet plan possible.

AI + DNA Testing for Hyper-Personalized Nutrition

No two bodies are the same, and genetics plays a major role in how we process nutrients, respond to exercise, and even experience hunger. Traditional diet plans treat everyone alike, but the next frontier is **hyper-personalized nutrition**: combining DNA insights with AI analysis to build nutrition strategies uniquely tailored to your biology.

By integrating genetic testing with AI platforms, individuals can receive guidance that goes beyond calories and macros — advice rooted in their own DNA. This means diet and supplement plans optimized for metabolism, food sensitivities, nutrient absorption, and even long-term disease risk.

How It Works

1. **DNA Analysis**
   - Genetic testing identifies markers tied to metabolism (e.g., lactose intolerance, caffeine sensitivity, fat processing efficiency).
2. **AI Integration**
   - AI combines genetic data with lifestyle inputs (diet, workouts, sleep) and biometric trends from wearables.
3. **Precision Recommendations**
   - Adjusts nutrition plans to align with genetic predispositions.
   - Suggests foods or supplements based on absorption efficiency and deficiencies.
4. **Long-Term Optimization**
   - Predicts how your genetic profile interacts with age, activity, and environmental factors to adapt plans over decades.

Why It Matters

- **Maximizes Efficiency**: Cuts trial and error by aligning diet with your biology.
- **Improves Safety**: Avoids foods or supplements your body struggles with.
- **Supports Longevity**: Addresses genetic risks before they impact health.
- **Creates Precision Health**: Moves from general guidelines to DNA-informed, data-driven nutrition.

Real-World Example

What Happened
A 37-year-old athlete constantly felt jittery on pre-workout formulas.

What Changed
DNA analysis revealed a genetic variation making him highly sensitive to caffeine. AI recalibrated his nutrition plan to remove caffeine and suggested L-theanine and adaptogens for focus instead.

Results
His performance improved, recovery stabilized, and anxiety dropped without sacrificing intensity.

What We Learn
Genetics often explains why "what works for others" doesn't always work for you.

Common Pitfalls

- **Over-Interpreting DNA**: Genes provide probabilities, not certainties.
- **Ignoring Lifestyle Factors**: DNA insights must be combined with behavior and environment.

- **Privacy Risks**: Genetic data is highly sensitive and must be securely stored.
- **Over-Supplementation**: DNA results can lead to unnecessary or excessive supplement use.

Tactical Best Practices

- **Pair DNA With Ongoing Tracking**: Combine genetics with AI-monitored lifestyle data.
- **Start With Food, Not Pills**: Use dietary adjustments before supplements.
- **Reassess Periodically**: Your genetics don't change, but lifestyle and environment do.
- **Choose Trusted Providers**: Use companies with strong data security policies.
- **Consult Professionals**: Pair AI insights with medical or nutritionist guidance for safety.

Final Thought

AI + DNA integration represents the cutting edge of personalized health. Instead of following generic plans, you'll follow a strategy written in your genetic code and adapted dynamically by AI to your lifestyle. This fusion promises the most individualized nutrition guidance ever created.

Next Steps
Beyond nutrition, the future of training is being reshaped by immersive technology. The next section explores **Virtual Reality + AI Workouts** — where interactive, adaptive training environments transform exercise into an engaging, data-driven experience.

Virtual Reality + AI Workouts

For decades, fitness routines have been bound by physical spaces —
gyms, studios, or living rooms. But the rise of **virtual reality (VR)
combined with AI** is breaking those walls down. Now, workouts
can take place in fully immersive environments where the scenery,
difficulty, and coaching adapt to you in real time.

Imagine boxing on a digital beach against an AI opponent that learns
your weaknesses, or running through a virtual mountain trail where
the incline and pace shift based on your heart rate. VR + AI
transforms workouts from repetitive tasks into engaging, gamified
experiences that keep motivation high and training personalized.

How VR + AI Workouts Function

1. **Immersive Environments**
   - Virtual landscapes keep exercise engaging and
     distract from fatigue.
2. **AI Adaptation**
   - The system adjusts intensity, form cues, and
     challenges based on your real-time performance and
     biometric feedback.
3. **Gamification**
   - Points, levels, and achievements keep users invested,
     similar to video games.
4. **Form & Safety Monitoring**
   - AI-powered motion tracking ensures proper form,
     reducing injury risk.
5. **Social Integration**
   - Multi-user VR environments allow group classes,
     competitions, and collaborative challenges.

Why This Matters

- **Increases Motivation**: Exercise feels like play, not punishment.
- **Improves Accessibility**: Brings world-class training into homes.
- **Enhances Safety**: Real-time feedback corrects form and intensity.
- **Expands Possibility**: Training no longer limited by space, weather, or equipment.

Real-World Example

What Happened
A 29-year-old found traditional cardio boring and inconsistent.

What Changed
She began VR-based cycling classes powered by AI, where the terrain and resistance adapted to her fitness levels. She also joined virtual group rides with friends across the globe.

Results
Her consistency skyrocketed, endurance improved, and she looked forward to workouts for the first time in years.

What We Learn
When exercise feels immersive and fun, adherence stops being the hardest part.

Common Pitfalls

- **Equipment Barriers**: VR headsets and sensors can be costly.
- **Overstimulation**: Some users may experience motion sickness or fatigue from immersive visuals.

- **Data Accuracy**: VR tracking may lag behind high-end wearables for precision metrics.
- **Isolation Risk**: Overuse of VR could reduce in-person social activity if not balanced.

Tactical Best Practices

- **Start Small**: Use VR workouts as a complement, not replacement, for traditional training.
- **Prioritize Safety**: Ensure adequate space and proper motion tracking.
- **Combine With Wearables**: Sync VR sessions with biometric data for accurate insights.
- **Seek Social Balance**: Use VR group classes to build community, not replace in-person interaction entirely.
- **Rotate Environments**: Prevent fatigue by exploring diverse virtual settings.

Final Thought

VR + AI represents the convergence of fitness, entertainment, and personalization. By making exercise immersive, adaptive, and socially connected, it has the potential to revolutionize how people experience movement — turning workouts into adventures rather than chores.

Next Steps
The immersive future doesn't stop at workouts. In the next section, we'll explore **AI-Driven Social Support Communities**, where digital platforms powered by intelligent systems create accountability, connection, and encouragement for long-term success.

AI-Driven Social Support Communities

One of the strongest predictors of long-term fitness and nutrition success isn't just the program you follow — it's the **people** you surround yourself with. Community provides accountability, encouragement, and a sense of belonging that fuels consistency. But traditional online groups or social media forums often lack personalization, making them hit-or-miss for genuine support.

AI is now powering a new wave of **intelligent social communities** that go beyond generic chatrooms. These platforms use machine learning to match individuals with peers, coaches, or mentors who share similar goals, struggles, and lifestyles. They also adapt over time, learning which types of interactions keep you most motivated and engaged.

How AI Shapes Social Fitness Communities

1. **Smart Matching**
   - Pairs users with accountability partners who have similar goals, schedules, or preferences.
2. **Personalized Challenges**
   - Creates group activities (step challenges, nutrition streaks, recovery check-ins) tailored to members' fitness levels.
3. **Sentiment & Engagement Analysis**
   - AI identifies when members lose motivation and nudges peers or moderators to provide encouragement.
4. **Global Connection**
   - Breaks geographic barriers, allowing support from a worldwide network of like-minded individuals.
5. **Toxicity Filtering**
   - AI moderates conversations to reduce misinformation, negativity, or unhealthy comparisons.

Why This Matters

- **Accountability**: Members are more likely to stick with routines when others cheer them on.
- **Belonging**: Reduces feelings of isolation in health journeys.
- **Sustained Motivation**: Social encouragement helps during inevitable dips in drive.
- **Collective Learning**: Members share strategies and experiences AI can further refine.

Real-World Example

What Happened
A 46-year-old office worker struggled to maintain consistency in solo training.

What Changed
He joined an AI-powered fitness community that matched him with three peers of similar age and goals. They participated in weekly walking challenges and shared meal prep ideas.

Results
He became more consistent with his steps, lost weight steadily, and reported higher motivation from the camaraderie.

What We Learn
Support tailored to your journey can make the difference between giving up and pushing through.

Common Pitfalls

- **Comparison Pressure**: Overemphasis on leaderboards can harm motivation if not balanced.
- **Superficial Engagement**: Communities that focus only on numbers may feel shallow.

- **Privacy Concerns**: Sharing progress or biometrics must be done securely.
- **Dependence on Community**: Over-reliance on external validation may hinder intrinsic motivation.

Tactical Best Practices

- **Choose Supportive Communities**: Look for groups moderated with empathy and inclusivity.
- **Set Shared but Flexible Goals**: Group targets should stretch members without creating unhealthy pressure.
- **Balance Social and Solo Work**: Use community for accountability, but nurture internal discipline.
- **Protect Your Privacy**: Limit what personal health details you share publicly.
- **Celebrate Collective Wins**: Focus on group encouragement, not just competition.

Final Thought

AI-driven social support communities combine the timeless power of human connection with the precision of intelligent technology. By curating the right networks, challenges, and encouragement, they transform fitness from a solitary task into a shared journey.

Next Steps
Beyond communities, the future of AI in fitness and nutrition lies in **Integration with Healthcare Systems** — bridging the gap between personal wellness tracking and professional medical care for a fully connected health ecosystem.

Integration with Healthcare Systems

Until now, fitness apps and healthcare systems have largely existed in silos. Your doctor might not see the detailed workout, nutrition, and sleep data you track daily, while your fitness platforms rarely integrate with clinical records. The future of health lies in closing this gap: **seamless integration between AI-powered fitness tools and professional healthcare systems.**

This integration will create a comprehensive view of health, where day-to-day wellness tracking informs clinical decisions, and medical insights shape personal fitness and nutrition strategies.

How Integration Could Work

1. **Unified Health Records**
   - Fitness, nutrition, and wearable data feed directly into your electronic health record (EHR).
   - Doctors gain real-time insights into your lifestyle outside of clinic visits.
2. **Preventive Care Alerts**
   - AI flags trends (e.g., rising blood pressure or declining sleep quality) and notifies both you and your physician.
3. **Personalized Treatment Plans**
   - Doctors prescribe exercise, diet, or supplementation guided by AI insights from your daily data.
4. **Remote Monitoring**
   - Patients with chronic conditions (diabetes, hypertension) can be monitored continuously, reducing hospital visits.
5. **Insurance & Wellness Incentives**
   - Healthcare providers and insurers may reward proactive behavior verified through AI-driven tracking.

Why This Matters

- **Holistic Care**: No more separation between "fitness goals" and "medical needs."
- **Earlier Interventions**: Doctors act before small problems escalate into major issues.
- **Better Compliance**: Patients follow advice more consistently when integrated with daily tools.
- **Reduced Costs**: Preventive care lowers long-term healthcare spending.

Real-World Example

What Happened
A 55-year-old with hypertension tracked his workouts, diet, and blood pressure via an AI app.

What Changed
His AI system synced with his doctor's EHR, automatically flagging irregular blood pressure trends. His physician adjusted medication and recommended stress-management practices before the condition worsened.

Results
He avoided hospitalization, improved lifestyle habits, and gained confidence knowing both his AI app and doctor were aligned.

What We Learn
When fitness data and medical care work together, prevention becomes practical, not just theoretical.

Common Pitfalls

- **Data Overload**: Doctors may struggle to process massive amounts of daily metrics without AI filtering.
- **Privacy Risks**: Sharing fitness data with healthcare networks increases exposure if not properly secured.

- **Equity Gaps**: Access to integrated systems may favor those with newer devices and higher incomes.
- **Over-Medicalization**: Risk of turning fitness into constant clinical oversight, reducing personal autonomy.

Tactical Best Practices

- **Seek Transparent Providers**: Work with apps that disclose how and if they share data with healthcare systems.
- **Prioritize Security**: Ensure data transfer between personal apps and medical systems is encrypted.
- **Set Boundaries**: Decide what data you're comfortable sharing with doctors.
- **Advocate for Simplicity**: Push for AI summaries (not raw data dumps) to aid doctors' decision-making.
- **Balance Autonomy and Care**: Use integration as support, not as surveillance.

Final Thought

Integration between AI health tools and medical systems represents the next great leap: a connected ecosystem where daily choices and clinical care reinforce each other. Done right, it will bridge the gap between fitness enthusiasts, healthcare providers, and prevention-focused medicine.

Next Steps
With integration shaping the near future, let's end with vision. In the final section, we'll explore **What the Next 10 Years May Look Like** — a forward-looking glimpse into how AI will transform the way we train, eat, recover, and live.

What the Next 10 Years May Look Like

The pace of innovation in AI-driven fitness and nutrition is accelerating, and the next decade will likely transform how we define health itself. What today feels futuristic — predictive disease prevention, hyper-personalized nutrition, immersive VR workouts — will become standard tools for everyday people. The coming years will be less about *if* these technologies emerge, and more about *how seamlessly they integrate into our lives.*

Key Predictions for the Next Decade

1. **From Tracking to Coaching**
   - AI will move beyond simply reporting data to becoming an adaptive health companion — offering moment-to-moment coaching, nudges, and adjustments tailored to your daily life.
2. **Healthcare + Fitness Convergence**
   - The line between personal wellness apps and clinical care will blur. Doctors, trainers, and AI platforms will share a single health ecosystem that covers prevention, treatment, and lifestyle management.
3. **DNA + Real-Time Biometrics**
   - Nutrition and training plans will combine genetic insights with daily biometrics, creating ultra-dynamic strategies that shift as your body changes.
4. **Immersive Training Environments**
   - VR and augmented reality (AR) will make workouts interactive, competitive, and globally social — turning fitness into a gamified, immersive experience accessible from home.
5. **AI-Driven Longevity**
   - Platforms will emphasize not just fitness goals, but extending healthspan — focusing on joint health, cognitive resilience, and disease prevention for aging populations.

6. **Regulation & Ethics Evolution**
    - o Stronger global laws will define who owns your data, how it's shared, and how safe AI health apps must be. Transparency will become a selling point, not an afterthought.
7. **Cultural Shift Toward Preventive Health**
    - o As AI makes prevention practical and accessible, societies will shift away from reactive healthcare models toward proactive, lifelong wellness strategies.

Real-World Glimpse

Consider a morning in 2035:

- Your wearable detects slightly elevated stress and reduced recovery from poor sleep.
- AI adjusts your workout plan to include mobility and meditation instead of heavy lifting.
- Breakfast is auto-suggested based on your glucose trends and genetic nutrient needs.
- A proactive message is sent to your healthcare provider flagging rising cholesterol markers, preventing a problem before it escalates.
- Later that evening, you join a global VR fitness challenge with friends across three continents, competing in real time with personalized coaching.

This isn't science fiction — it's the logical progression of technologies already in motion.

Common Pitfalls to Avoid

- **Over-Automation**: The risk of letting AI control health entirely, sidelining human judgment.
- **Equity Gaps**: Access to advanced tools may initially favor wealthier populations, widening health divides.

- **Data Overreach**: Without safeguards, personal health data could become a commodity instead of a protected right.
- **Lifestyle Over-Quantification**: Reducing health to numbers while losing sight of enjoyment and intuition.

Tactical Advice for the Future

- **Stay Adaptive**: Embrace new tools but remain critical of their promises.
- **Prioritize Security**: Treat your health data as valuable property.
- **Use AI as a Partner**: Let technology guide and simplify, but keep self-awareness central.
- **Focus on Healthspan**: Look beyond short-term goals to the habits that sustain lifelong vitality.
- **Advocate for Access**: Push for ethical and inclusive AI health solutions across all demographics.

Final Thought

The next 10 years will redefine what it means to take care of yourself. Fitness and nutrition will no longer be fragmented or reactive but **integrated, predictive, and deeply personal.** AI will act as both a coach and a safeguard, helping people not only reach their goals but live longer, healthier, and more empowered lives.

The future is not about replacing human wisdom with machines — it's about combining the two. When AI's intelligence meets human intuition, the result is a world where health isn't just managed, but mastered.

Glossary of Key Terms

This glossary provides clear, practical definitions of important terms used throughout the book. Each entry is explained in plain language for fitness enthusiasts, professionals, and decision-makers who want to understand both the technical and practical sides of AI in health.

A

AI (Artificial Intelligence)
Computer systems designed to mimic human learning, reasoning, and decision-making. In fitness and nutrition, AI analyzes large amounts of data to create personalized plans, detect patterns, and provide recommendations.

AI Coaching Apps
Mobile or web-based platforms that use AI to deliver personalized workout, diet, and motivational guidance.

AI Nudges
Timely reminders or prompts generated by AI, encouraging healthy behavior like drinking water, logging meals, or getting more sleep.

Algorithmic Bias
When an AI system produces unfair or inaccurate outcomes due to biased data or flawed design.

Augmented Reality (AR)
Technology that overlays digital elements (e.g., workout cues, stats) onto real-world environments through glasses or phone screens.

B

Biomarkers
Measurable biological signals such as heart rate, blood glucose, or hormone levels that provide insights into health and performance.

Biofeedback
The use of real-time data (like heart rate variability) to monitor and improve physical or mental performance.

C

Calories In vs. Calories Out
The principle of energy balance: weight change is influenced by the calories you consume versus the calories you burn.

Carbon Tracking
In nutrition apps, a feature that measures the environmental impact of food choices — sometimes integrated into AI diet planners.

Circadian Rhythm
The body's natural 24-hour cycle regulating sleep, energy, and hormone release, which AI often considers when recommending training or nutrition timing.

Continuous Glucose Monitoring (CGM)
Wearable sensors that track blood sugar in real time. AI interprets this data to guide meal timing and food choices.

D

Data Privacy
The protection of personal health information collected by apps, wearables, or healthcare systems.

Deficiency Prediction
AI's ability to forecast nutrient shortfalls before they cause symptoms, based on diet logs and lifestyle data.

DNA Testing
Genetic analysis that reveals predispositions for nutrient absorption, exercise response, or health risks.

E

Energy Balance
The equilibrium between calories consumed and calories expended. Central to weight management and performance.

Ethical AI
AI systems designed with transparency, fairness, and privacy protections to ensure responsible use of health data.

EHR (Electronic Health Record)
A digital version of a patient's medical history, which may one day integrate with AI fitness platforms.

F

Feedback Loop
The process of AI adjusting recommendations based on user behavior and outcomes. For example, altering a diet plan after logging food consistently for two weeks.

Form Correction (AI Video Analysis)
Computer vision technology that analyzes exercise technique in real time and provides adjustments to reduce injury risk.

G

Gamification
The use of points, levels, or rewards in apps to make fitness and nutrition feel more engaging.

Gut Microbiome
The community of bacteria and microorganisms in the digestive tract that affects nutrient absorption, energy, immunity, and mood.

H

Healthspan
The portion of life spent in good health, free from chronic disease or disability. AI tools increasingly aim to extend healthspan, not just lifespan.

HRV (Heart Rate Variability)
A measure of the variation in time between heartbeats, often used to assess stress and recovery.

Hyper-Personalized Nutrition
Tailoring diet plans to an individual's DNA, biometrics, and lifestyle through AI-driven analysis.

I

Intuitive Eating
An approach to nutrition focused on listening to hunger and fullness cues rather than rigid tracking. AI may integrate these cues into flexible guidance.

Integration
The connection of AI health apps with medical systems, creating unified care between personal wellness and professional healthcare.

L

Longevity
The length of a person's life. In this book, longevity focuses on increasing not just years lived but years lived in good health.

M

Macronutrients (Macros)
Nutrients required in large amounts: proteins, fats, and

carbohydrates. AI tools often optimize their balance for performance or weight goals.

Micronutrients
Vitamins and minerals required in smaller amounts but essential for health. AI helps detect and address gaps in intake.

Motion Tracking
Technology that records movement patterns during exercise, often used by AI for form correction.

N

Nutrient Timing
Aligning meals and supplements with activity and recovery windows to maximize performance. AI optimizes this based on workouts, sleep, and biometrics.

P

Pattern Recognition
AI's ability to identify repeated habits or behaviors (e.g., overeating at night, skipping workouts on Fridays).

Predictive Modeling
AI techniques that forecast future outcomes, such as plateaus, nutrient deficiencies, or disease risks.

Privacy Breach
An incident where personal health data is accessed or shared without permission.

R

Readiness Score
A metric generated by wearables and AI that indicates how prepared your body is for exercise, based on sleep, stress, and recovery data.

Recovery Tracking
Monitoring sleep, HRV, and other data to determine how well the body is healing from training.

S

Sleep Hygiene
Daily habits and routines that promote quality sleep. AI often suggests improvements based on tracked sleep data.

Smart Wearables
Devices like watches, rings, or patches that monitor biometrics and sync data with AI platforms.

Supplementation
The use of vitamins, minerals, or performance aids to fill dietary gaps. AI helps personalize choices and dosages.

T

Tracking Fatigue
Burnout from excessive self-monitoring, often linked to disordered eating or exercise obsession.

Transparency
The obligation for AI apps and companies to clearly explain how data is collected, stored, and used.

V

Virtual Reality (VR) Workouts
Immersive training experiences where users exercise in simulated environments. When combined with AI, VR adapts workouts in real time.

W

Wearable Data Integration
Combining multiple devices (smartwatches, glucose monitors, sleep trackers) into one AI system for a unified health picture.

Wellness Ecosystem
The interconnected system of fitness, nutrition, mental health, and medical care — increasingly integrated by AI.

Thank you for taking the time to read this Book.

If you found value in this book, I'd be deeply grateful if you took a few minutes of your time to share your feedback. An **honnest review on Amazon**, a personal recommendation to a colleague, or simply applying what you've learned in your work all go a long way. Your encouragement helps fuel future writing, research, and tool development — and inspires continued work that makes a real difference in the community.

— Eric LeBouthillier
Founder, AcraSolution

www.ingramcontent.com/pod-product-compliance
Lightning Source LLC
Chambersburg PA
CBHW062123020426
42335CB00013B/1076